Patient Safety and Quality Improvement

Editor

RAHUL K. SHAH

OTOLARYNGOLOGIC CLINICS OF NORTH AMERICA

www.oto.theclinics.com

Consulting Editor
SUJANA S. CHANDRASEKHAR

February 2019 • Volume 52 • Number 1

ELSEVIER

1600 John F. Kennedy Boulevard • Suite 1800 • Philadelphia, Pennsylvania, 19103-2899

http://www.oto.theclinics.com

OTOLARYNGOLOGIC CLINICS OF NORTH AMERICA Volume 52, Number 1
February 2019 ISSN 0030-6665, ISBN-13: 978-0-323-65481-4

Editor: Jessica McCool
Developmental Editor: Sara Watkins

Otolaryngologic Clinics of North America (ISSN 0030-6665) is published bimonthly by Elsevier, Inc., 360 Park Avenue South, New York, NY 10010-1710. Months of issue are February, April, June, August, October, and December. Business and Editorial Offices: 1600 John F. Kennedy Blvd., Suite 1800, Philadelphia, PA 19103-2899. Customer Service Office: 6277 Sea Harbor Drive, Orlando, FL 32887-4800. Periodicals postage paid at New York, NY and additional mailing offices. Subscription prices are $412.00 per year (US individuals), $889.00 per year (US institutions), $100.00 per year (US student/resident), $548.00 per year (Canadian individuals), $1127.00 per year (Canadian institutions), $564.00 per year (international individuals), $1127.00 per year (international institutions), $270.00 per year (international & Canadian student/resident). Foreign air speed delivery is included in all *Clinics'* subscription prices. All prices are subject to change without notice. **POSTMASTER:** Send address changes to *Otolaryngologic Clinics of North America*, Elsevier Health Sciences Division, Subscription Customer Service, 3251 Riverport Lane, Maryland Heights, MO 63043. **Telephone: 1-800-654-2452 (U.S. and Canada); 314-447-8871 (outside U.S. and Canada). Fax: 314-447-8029. E-mail: journalscustomerservice-usa@elsevier.com (for print support); journalsonlinesupport-usa@elsevier.com (for online support).**

Reprints. For copies of 100 or more of articles in this publication, please contact the Commercial Reprints Department, Elsevier Inc., 360 Park Avenue South, New York, NY 10010-1710. Tel.: 212-633-3874; Fax: 212-633-3820; E-mail: reprints@elsevier.com.

Otolaryngologic Clinics of North America is also published in Spanish by McGraw-Hill Interamericana Editores S.A., P.O. Box 5-237, 06500 Mexico D.F., Mexico.

Otolaryngologic Clinics of North America is covered in *MEDLINE/PubMed (Index Medicus), Current Contents/Clinical Medicine, Excerpta Medica, BIOSIS, Science Citation Index,* and *ISI/BIOMED.*

PROGRAM OBJECTIVE

The goal of the *Otolaryngologic Clinics of North America* is to provide information on the latest trends in patient management, the newest advances; and provide a sound basis for choosing treatment options in the field of otolaryngology.

LEARNING OBJECTIVES

Upon completion of this activity, participants will be able to:

1. Review best practices in medical device safety and standards
2. Discuss best practices to improve quality of care for tracheostomy patients
3. Recognize patient safety and quality office-based procedures in Otolaryngology

ACCREDITATION

The Elsevier Office of Continuing Medical Education (EOCME) is accredited by the Accreditation Council for Continuing Medical Education (ACCME) to provide continuing medical education for physicians.

The EOCME designates this enduring material for a maximum of 15 *AMA PRA Category 1 Credit*(s)™. Physicians should claim only the credit commensurate with the extent of their participation in the activity.

All other health care professionals requesting continuing education credit for this enduring material will be issued a certificate of participation.

DISCLOSURE OF CONFLICTS OF INTEREST

The EOCME assesses conflict of interest with its instructors, faculty, planners, and other individuals who are in a position to control the content of CME activities. All relevant conflicts of interest that are identified are thoroughly vetted by EOCME for fair balance, scientific objectivity, and patient care recommendations. EOCME is committed to providing its learners with CME activities that promote improvements or quality in healthcare and not a specific proprietary business or a commercial interest.

The planning committee, staff, authors and editors listed below have identified no financial relationships or relationships to products or devices they or their spouse/life partner have with commercial interest related to the content of this CME activity:

Tracey Ambrose, AuD, CCC-A; Ellis M. Arjmand, MD, MMM, PhD; Christine L. Barron, BA; Joshua R. Bedwell, MD, MS, FAAP, FACS; Emily F. Boss, MD, MPH; Sarah N. Bowe, MD; Michael J. Brenner, MD, FACS; Richard J. Brilli, MD; Tanis S. Cameron, MA-SLP (C) CCC-SLP; Sujana S. Chandrasekhar, MD, FACS, FAAOHNS; C.W. David Chang, MD, FACS; Silas Chao, BS; Richard A. Chole, MD, PhD; Wallace Crandall, MD, MMM; Ellen S. Deutsch, MD, MS, FACS, FAAP; Alexandra G. Espinel, MD; Lyuba Gitman, MD; Stacey T. Gray, MD; Ian N. Jacobs, MD; Alison Kemp; Elliana R. Kirsh, BM, BS; Mimi S. Kokoska, MD, MHCM, FACS, CPE; Jennifer M. Lavin, MD, MS; Stephanie Lemle, MBA; Toby Litovitz, MD; Jessica McCool; Michael E. McCormick, MD; Brendan A. McGrath, MBChB, MRCP, FRCA, DICM, EDIC, PGCertMedEd, AHEA, FFICM, PhD; Erin L. McKean, MD, MBA; Lemmietta G. McNeilly, PhD, CCC-SLP; Brian Nussenbaum, MD, MHCM; Mary D. Patterson, MD, MEd; Vinay K. Rathi, MD; Srijaya K. Reddy, MD, MBA; David W. Roberson, MD, MBA, FACS, FRCS; Tommie L. Robinson, Jr, PhD, CCC-SLP, FASHA, FNAP; Soham Roy, MD, FACS, FAAP; Marisa A. Ryan, MD, MPH; Alexander L. Schneider, MD; Prerak D. Shah, MD, FACS; Rahul K. Shah, MD, MBA; Emily K. Shuman, MD; Lee P. Smith, MD, FACS, FAAP; Carl H. Snyderman, MD, MBA; Subhalakshmi Vaidyanathan; Andrew T. Waberski, MD; Sara Watkins.

The planning committee, staff, authors and editors listed below have identified financial relationships or relationships to products or devices they or their spouse/life partner have with commercial interest related to the content of this CME activity:

Karthik Balakrishnan, MD, MPH: receives research support from Rosivo Inc.

Charles A. Elmaraghy, MD: holds a patent with Marpac, Inc. and serves as a consultant/advisor to Smith & Nephew.

Kris R. Jatana, MD: is a consultant/advisor for Intertek Group plc and holds a patent with Marpac, Inc.

Vinciya Pandian, PhD, MBA, MSN, RN, ACNP-BC, FAAN: is a consultant/advisor for Medtronic and receives research support from Smiths Medical.

UNAPPROVED/OFF-LABEL USE DISCLOSURE

The EOCME requires CME faculty to disclose to the participants:

1. When products or procedures being discussed are off-label, unlabelled, experimental, and/or investigational (not US Food and Drug Administration [FDA] approved); and

2. Any limitations on the information presented, such as data that are preliminary or that represent ongoing research, interim analyses, and/or unsupported opinions. Faculty may discuss information about pharmaceutical agents that is outside of FDA-approved labelling. This information is intended solely for CME and is not intended to promote off-label use of these medications. If you have any questions, contact the medical affairs department of the manufacturer for the most recent prescribing information.

TO ENROLL
To enroll in the *Otolaryngologic Clinics of North America* Continuing Medical Education program, call customer service at 1-800-654-2452 or sign up online at http://www.theclinics.com/home/cme. The CME program is available to subscribers for an additional annual fee of USD 260.

METHOD OF PARTICIPATION
In order to claim credit, participants must complete the following:
1. Complete enrolment as indicated above.
2. Read the activity.
3. Complete the CME Test and Evaluation. Participants must achieve a score of 70% on the test. All CME Tests and Evaluations must be completed online.

CME INQUIRIES/SPECIAL NEEDS
For all CME inquiries or special needs, please contact elsevierCME@elsevier.com.

Contributors

CONSULTING EDITOR

SUJANA S. CHANDRASEKHAR, MD, FACS, FAAOHNS
Past President, American Academy of Otolaryngology–Head and Neck Surgery, Partner, ENT & Allergy Associates, LLP, Clinical Professor, Department of Otolaryngology–Head and Neck Surgery, Zucker School of Medicine at Hofstra-Northwell, Hempstead, New York; Clinical Associate Professor, Department of Otolaryngology–Head and Neck Surgery, Icahn School of Medicine at Mount Sinai, New York, New York, USA

EDITOR

RAHUL K. SHAH, MD, MBA
Vice President, Chief Quality and Safety Officer, Professor of Otolaryngology and Pediatrics, Children's National Health System, George Washington University School of Medicine and Health Sciences, Washington, DC, USA

AUTHORS

TRACEY AMBROSE, AuD, CCC-A
Lead Audiologist, Division of Hearing and Speech, Children's National Health System, Washington, DC, USA

ELLIS M. ARJMAND, MD, MMM, PhD
Bobby Alford Department of Otolaryngology–Head and Neck Surgery, Texas Children's Hospital, Baylor College of Medicine, Houston, Texas, USA

KARTHIK BALAKRISHNAN, MD, MPH
Department of Otorhinolaryngology, Mayo Clinic Children's Center, Mayo Clinic College of Medicine and Science, Rochester, Minnesota, USA

CHRISTINE L. BARRON, BA
The Ohio State University College of Medicine, Columbus, Ohio, USA

JOSHUA R. BEDWELL, MD, MS, FAAP, FACS
Associate Professor, Department of Otolaryngology, Texas Children's Hospital, Baylor College of Medicine, Houston, Texas, USA

EMILY F. BOSS, MD, MPH
Associate Professor of Otolaryngology–Head and Neck Surgery, Pediatrics, and Health Policy and Management, Director, Pediatric Surgical Quality and Safety, Bloomberg Children's Center, Johns Hopkins University School of Medicine and Bloomberg School of Public Health, Baltimore, Maryland, USA

SARAH N. BOWE, MD
Assistant Professor, Department of Otolaryngology–Head and Neck Surgery, San Antonio Uniformed Services Health Education Consortium, JBSA-Fort Sam Houston, Texas, USA

MICHAEL J. BRENNER, MD, FACS
Associate Professor, Department of Otolaryngology–Head and Neck Surgery, University of Michigan School of Medicine, Ann Arbor, Michigan, USA

RICHARD J. BRILLI, MD
Division of Pediatric Critical Care Medicine, Department of Pediatrics, The Ohio State University College of Medicine, Nationwide Children's Hospital, Columbus, Ohio, USA

TANIS S. CAMERON, MA-SLP (C) CCC-SLP
Austin Health, Heidelberg, Victoria, Australia

C.W. DAVID CHANG, MD, FACS
Jerry W. Templer, MD, Faculty Scholar, Associate Clinical Professor of Otolaryngology, Department of Otolaryngology–Head and Neck Surgery, University of Missouri School of Medicine, Columbia, Missouri, USA

SILAS CHAO, BS
Northeast Ohio Medical University, Rootstown, Ohio, USA

RICHARD A. CHOLE, MD, PhD
Professor, Department of Otolaryngology, Washington University in St Louis, School of Medicine, St Louis, Missouri, USA

WALLACE CRANDALL, MD, MMM
Quality Improvement Services, Division of Pediatric Gastroenterology, Hepatology, and Nutrition, Department of Pediatrics, The Ohio State University College of Medicine, Nationwide Children's Hospital, Columbus, Ohio, USA

ELLEN S. DEUTSCH, MD, MS, FACS, FAAP
Medical Director, Pennsylvania Patient Safety Authority, Harrisburg, Pennsylvania, USA; ECRI Institute, Plymouth Meeting, Pennsylvania, USA; Adjunct Associate Professor, Senior Scientist, Department of Anesthesiology and Critical Care Medicine, University of Pennsylvania Perelman School of Medicine, Philadelphia, Pennsylvania, USA

CHARLES A. ELMARAGHY, MD
Department of Pediatric Otolaryngology, Nationwide Children's Hospital, Department of Otolaryngology–Head and Neck Surgery, The Ohio State University Wexner Medical Center, Columbus, Ohio, USA

ALEXANDRA G. ESPINEL, MD
Assistant Professor, Otolaryngology and Pediatrics, Division of Otolaryngology, Children's National Health System, George Washington University School of Medicine and Health Sciences, Washington, DC, USA

LYUBA GITMAN, MD
Assistant Professor, Pediatrics, Division of ENT, Children's National Health System, George Washington University School of Medicine and Health Sciences, Washington, DC, USA

STACEY T. GRAY, MD
Associate Professor, Department of Otolaryngology–Head and Neck Surgery, Massachusetts Eye and Ear Infirmary; Department of Otolaryngology, Harvard Medical School, Boston, Massachusetts, USA

IAN N. JACOBS, MD
Division of Pediatric Otolaryngology, Children's Hospital of Philadelphia, Department of Otorhinolaryngology–Head and Neck Surgery, University of Pennsylvania Perelman School of Medicine, Philadelphia, Pennsylvania, USA

KRIS R. JATANA, MD
Department of Pediatric Otolaryngology, Nationwide Children's Hospital, Department of Otolaryngology–Head and Neck Surgery, The Ohio State University Wexner Medical Center, Columbus, Ohio, USA

ELLIANA R. KIRSH, BM, BS
Harvard Medical School, Brookline, Massachusetts, USA

MIMI S. KOKOSKA, MD, MHCM, FACS, CPE
Senior Vice President, Strategic Partnerships and Innovation, Healthcare Quality and Affordability, Blue Shield of California, San Francisco, California, USA

JENNIFER M. LAVIN, MD, MS
Department of Otolaryngology–Head and Neck Surgery, Northwestern University, Northwestern Memorial Hospital, Division of Pediatric Otolaryngology–Head and Neck Surgery, Ann and Robert H. Lurie Children's Hospital of Chicago, Chicago, Illinois, USA

STEPHANIE LEMLE, MBA
Quality Improvement Services, Nationwide Children's Hospital, Columbus, Ohio, USA

TOBY LITOVITZ, MD
National Capital Poison Center, Washington, DC, USA

MICHAEL E. McCORMICK, MD
Associate Professor, Department of Otolaryngology and Communication Sciences, Medical College of Wisconsin, Milwaukee, Wisconsin

BRENDAN A. McGRATH, MBChB, MRCP, FRCA, DICM, EDIC, PGCertMedEd, AHEA, FFICM, PhD
Consultant in Anaesthesia and Intensive Care Medicine, Manchester University Hospital NHS Foundation Trust, Honorary Senior Lecturer, Division of Infection, Immunity and Respiratory Medicine, Faculty of Biology, Medicine and Health, The University of Manchester, Wythenshawe, Manchester, United Kingdom

ERIN L. McKEAN, MD, MBA
Associate Professor, Otolaryngology–Head and Neck Surgery and Neurosurgery, University of Michigan, Ann Arbor, Michigan, USA

LEMMIETTA G. McNEILLY, PhD, CCC-SLP
Chief Staff Officer, Speech-Language Pathology, American Speech-Language-Hearing Association, Rockville, Maryland, USA

BRIAN NUSSENBAUM, MD, MHCM
Executive Director, American Board of Otolaryngology, Houston, Texas, USA

VINCIYA PANDIAN, PhD, MBA, MSN, RN, ACNP-BC, FAAN
Assistant Professor, Acute and Chronic Care, Johns Hopkins School of Nursing, Baltimore, Maryland, USA

MARY D. PATTERSON, MD, MEd
Associate Dean of Experiential Learning, Center for Experiential Learning and Simulation, Professor of Emergency Medicine, University of Florida, Gainesville, Florida, USA

VINAY K. RATHI, MD
Resident Physician, Department of Otolaryngology–Head and Neck Surgery, Massachusetts Eye and Ear Infirmary; Department of Otolaryngology, Harvard Medical School, Boston, Massachusetts, USA

SRIJAYA K. REDDY, MD, MBA
Associate Professor of Anesthesiology, Division of Pediatric Anesthesiology, Monroe Carell Jr Children's Hospital at Vanderbilt, Vanderbilt University School of Medicine, Nashville, Tennessee, USA

DAVID W. ROBERSON, MD, MBA, FACS, FRCS
President, The Global Tracheostomy Collaborative, West Roxbury, Massachusetts, USA

TOMMIE L. ROBINSON Jr, PhD, CCC-SLP, FASHA, FNAP
Chief, Division of Hearing and Speech, Director, Scottish Rite Center for Childhood Language Disorders, Associate Professor, Pediatrics, Children's National Health System, Scottish Rite Center for Childhood Language Disorders, George Washington University School of Medicine and Health Sciences, Washington, DC, USA

SOHAM ROY, MD, FACS, FAAP
Professor and Chief, Pediatric Otolaryngology, Department of Otorhinolaryngology, University of Texas at Houston McGovern Medical School, Houston, Texas, USA

MARISA A. RYAN, MD, MPH
Instructor of Otolaryngology–Head and Neck Surgery, Department of Otolaryngology, Head and Neck Surgery, Johns Hopkins University School of Medicine, Baltimore, Maryland, USA

ALEXANDER L. SCHNEIDER, MD
Department of Otolaryngology–Head and Neck Surgery, Northwestern University Feinberg School of Medicine, Chicago, Illinois, USA

PRERAK D. SHAH, MD, FACS
New England Ear, Nose and Throat Center & Facial Plastic Surgery, Clinical Instructor, Harvard Medical School, Associate Surgeon, Massachusetts Eye and Ear Infirmary, North Andover, Massachusetts, USA

EMILY K. SHUMAN, MD
Assistant Professor of Internal Medicine, Division of Infectious Diseases, University of Michigan Medical School, Ann Arbor, Michigan, USA

LEE P. SMITH, MD, FACS, FAAP
Associate Professor, Department of Otolaryngology, Hofstra Northwell School of Medicine, Chief of Pediatric Otolaryngology, Cohen Children's Medical Center, Northwell Health, Northwell Health System, Queens, New York, USA

CARL H. SNYDERMAN, MD, MBA
Professor, Departments of Otolaryngology and Neurological Surgery, University of Pittsburgh School of Medicine, The Eye & Ear Institute, Pittsburgh, Pennsylvania, USA

ANDREW T. WABERSKI, MD
Assistant Professor of Anesthesiology and Pediatrics, Division of Anesthesiology, Pain and Perioperative Medicine, Children's National Health System, George Washington University School of Medicine and Health Sciences, Washington, DC, USA

Contents

Foreword: Delivering Otolaryngologic Care Safely and Successfully xv

Sujana S. Chandrasekhar

Preface: Patient Safety and Quality Improvement: Driving to New Frontiers xix

Rahul K. Shah

Systems Science: A Primer on High Reliability 1

David W. Roberson and Elliana R. Kirsh

> In the 21st century, most medical care is not delivered by a single physician but rather, by a team. A team is a type of system, a set of people and things interacting together for a defined aim. The discipline of systems science concerns itself with how complex teams or organizations function. The application of systems science has had a major positive impact on safety and quality in such diverse disciplines as auto manufacturing, airline safety, and nuclear power generation. A modest understanding of how systems science applies to medical care can help improve safety and quality of care.

Leadership Driving Safety and Quality 11

Erin L. McKean and Carl H. Snyderman

> Leaders in health care play a large role in successful achievement of quality and safety goals through an overt commitment to both quality and safety, fostering a culture of quality improvement and clear and consistent communication of goals and plans. Specific training for frontline providers, managers, and staff is critical in developing skilled leaders with a quality and safety orientation. Many models exist for organizational leadership development, and exemplars of quality and safety leadership have openly shared the keys to their successes for others to raise the bar.

Patient Engagement in Otolaryngology 23

Marisa A. Ryan and Emily F. Boss

> Patient engagement, which involves incorporating the patient and family as partners in their care, is a growing focus in otolaryngology and surgery. Attention to patient and family centeredness, shared decision making, and patient experience together improves the overall tenor of patient engagement. Patient engagement promotes safety through improving quality of electronic health record data, error detection, and treatment decisions and adherence. In this article, we review specific areas of importance for patient engagement in otolaryngology as well as areas needing more research and development.

The Impact of Cognitive and Implicit Bias on Patient Safety and Quality   35

Karthik Balakrishnan and Ellis M. Arjmand

> Humans use cognitive shortcuts, or heuristics, to quickly assess and respond to situations and data. When applied inappropriately, heuristics have the potential to redirect analysis of available information in consistent ways, creating systematic biases resulting in decision errors. Heuristics have greater effect in high-pressure, high-stakes decisions, particularly when dealing with incomplete information, in other words, daily medical and surgical practice. This article discusses 2 major categories: cognitive biases, which affect how we perceive and interpret clinical data; and implicit biases, which affect how we perceive and respond to other individuals, and also discusses approaches to recognize and alleviate bias effects.

Rethinking Morbidity and Mortality Conference   47

Brian Nussenbaum and Richard A. Chole

> This article will discuss the importance of an effective morbidity and mortality (M&M) conference toward supporting a proactive and preventative approach to patient safety and quality improvement (PSQI). Key characteristics will be discussed that enhance this process for being a mechanism for driving positive PSQI culture change that permeates the department. The focus of this article will be on how to approach the structure and process of this conference for maximal benefit.

Resident and Fellow Engagement in Safety and Quality   55

Sarah N. Bowe and Michael E. McCormick

> Beyond educational and institutional requirements, there is a need for trainees (residents and fellows) to learn patient safety and quality improvement skills in order to achieve the ultimate goal of providing better patient care. Key steps to engagement include creating a safety and quality culture, supporting faculty development, and selecting appropriate curricular resources. Efforts to align the goals and processes of the graduate medical education institution and teaching hospital can foster a unified mission. Faculty must be prepared to teach and reinforce these topics on a regular basis. Both didactic instruction and experiential learning are necessary components for trainee education.

Anesthesia Safety in Otolaryngology   63

Andrew T. Waberski, Alexandra G. Espinel, and Srijaya K. Reddy

> This article highlights the important relationship between the otolaryngologist and anesthesiologist, focusing on intraoperative patient safety for otolaryngologic surgery. In addition, consideration of preoperative history, physical examination, and potential postoperative complications helps guide the otolaryngologist and anesthesiologist in formulating an appropriate and collaborative management strategy.

Patient Safety in Audiology   **75**

Tommie L. Robinson Jr, Tracey Ambrose, Lyuba Gitman, and
Lemmietta G. McNeilly

There is a need to educate audiologists, physicians, and other clinicians about patient safety in audiology. This article addresses the many aspects of patient safety and the applicability to the practice of audiology in health care. Clinical examples of strategies to build a culture of patient safety are provided.

Patient Safety and Quality for Office-Based Procedures in Otolaryngology   **89**

Prerak D. Shah

Office-based procedures have increased in frequency with the recent changes in the current health care climate prioritizing improved efficiency and greater value in the care that is delivered. This article focuses on patient safety and quality issues that are specific to procedures in the office setting of an Otolaryngologist. Specific topics are categorized into preprocedure planning, procedural execution, and postprocedure follow-up. Several best practice recommendations are included to promote and simplify the integration of these quality and safety measures into every office setting.

Device Safety   **103**

Vinay K. Rathi and Stacey T. Gray

Medical devices are essential in the diagnosis and treatment of otolaryngologic disease. The US Food and Drug Administration (FDA) is tasked with assuring the safety and effectiveness of these devices. Otolaryngologists, in turn, are often responsible for helping patients understand risks, benefits, and alternatives when deciding whether to rely on devices in their care. To best counsel patients, otolaryngologists should be aware of the strengths and limitations of device regulation by the FDA. This article reviews the FDA regulatory framework for medical devices, premarket evidentiary standards for marketing devices, and postmarket methods of safety surveillance.

Simulation Saves the Day (and Patient)   **115**

Ellen S. Deutsch and Mary D. Patterson

Surgeons can use simulation to improve the safety of the systems they work within, around, because of, and despite. Health care is a complex adaptive system that can never be completely knowable; simulation can expose aspects of patient care delivery that are not necessarily evident prospectively, during planning, or retrospectively, during investigations or audits. The constraints of patient care processes and adaptive capacity of health care providers may become most evident during simulations conducted "in situ" using real teams and real equipment, in actual patient care locations.

Clinical Indices to Drive Quality Improvement in Otolaryngology   **123**

Christine L. Barron, Charles A. Elmaraghy, Stephanie Lemle,
Wallace Crandall, Richard J. Brilli, and Kris R. Jatana

A Pediatric Tracheostomy Care Index (PTCI) was developed by the authors to standardize care and drive quality improvement efforts at their institution. The PTCI comprises 9 elements deemed essential for safe care of children with a tracheostomy tube. Based on the PTCI scores, the number of missed opportunities per patient was tracked, and interventions through a "Plan-Do-Study-Act" approach were performed. The establishment of the PTCI has been successful at standardizing, quantifying, and monitoring the consistency and documentation of care provided at the authors' institution.

Multidisciplinary Tracheostomy Care: How Collaboratives Drive Quality Improvement   135

Joshua R. Bedwell, Vinciya Pandian, David W. Roberson, Brendan A. McGrath, Tanis S. Cameron, and Michael J. Brenner

There have been reports of successful quality-improvement initiatives surrounding tracheostomy care for more than a decade, but widespread adoption of best practices has not been universal. Five key drivers have been found to improve the quality of care for tracheostomy patients: multidisciplinary synchronous ward rounds, standardization of care protocols, appropriate interdisciplinary education and staff allocation, patient and family involvement, and use of data to drive improvement. The Global Tracheostomy Collaborative is a quality-improvement collaborative dedicated to improving the care of tracheostomy patients worldwide through communication, dissemination, and implementation of proven strategies based on these 5 key drivers.

Button Battery Safety: Industry and Academic Partnerships to Drive Change   149

Kris R. Jatana, Silas Chao, Ian N. Jacobs, and Toby Litovitz

The pediatric button battery (BB) hazard has been recognized for several decades. In 2012, the National Button Battery Task Force was established, and most manufacturers have improved warning labels, more secure packaging, and made BB compartments in products are more secure. Tissue neutralization before BB removal (ie, honey or sucralfate/Carafate®) is an effective way to reduce the rate of BB injury. In absence of visible perforation, 0.25% sterile acetic acid esophageal tissue irrigation at time of BB removal is recommended as a neutralization strategy to mitigate injury progression. Future BB design changes could eliminate esophageal tissue injury.

Preventing and Managing Operating Room Fires in Otolaryngology—Head and Neck Surgery   163

Soham Roy and Lee P. Smith

Otolaryngologists are at high risk of surgical fire. During surgery in the head and neck region there is close proximity of 3 essential elements: an ignition source, a fuel, and an oxidizing agent. In this article, the authors highlight the scenarios where fire may occur and offer steps that surgeons can take to minimize risk for their patients. By understanding the elements of the fire triad, otolaryngologists can decrease the risk of surgical fire, through careful control of oxidizers, ignition sources, and potential fuels in the operating room.

Reprocessing Standards for Medical Devices and Equipment in Otolaryngology: Safe Practices for Scopes, Speculums, and Single-Use Devices   **173**

C.W. David Chang, Michael J. Brenner, Emily K. Shuman, and Mimi S. Kokoska

Stringent regulatory standards for reprocessing medical devices and equipment have proliferated in response to patient safety incidents in which improperly disinfected or contaminated endoscopes lead to large-scale disease transmission or outbreaks. This article details best practices in reprocessing reusable and single-use devices in otolaryngology, with particular attention to flexible fiberoptic endoscopes/nasophyarngoscopes, nasal speculums, and other clinic and operating room instruments. High-risk devices require sterilization, whereas lower risk devices may be reprocessed using various disinfection procedures. Reprocessing practices have implications for adequacy, efficiency, and cost. Nuanced understanding of procedures and their rationale ensures delivery of safe, ethical, and quality patient care.

Publicly Available Databases in Otolaryngology Quality Improvement   **185**

Alexander L. Schneider and Jennifer M. Lavin

The historical context for quality improvement is provided. Important differences are described between the two overarching types of databases: clinical registries and administrative databases. The pros and cons of each are provided as are examples of their utilization in otolaryngology–head and neck surgery.

OTOLARYNGOLOGIC CLINICS OF NORTH AMERICA

FORTHCOMING ISSUES

April 2019
Implantable Auditory Devices
Darius Kohan and
Sujana S. Chandrasekhar, *Editors*

June 2019
Office-Based Surgery in Otolaryngology
Melissa Pynnonen and Cecelia
Schmalbach, *Editors*

August 2019
Advancements in Clinical Laryngology
Jonathan M. Bock, Chandra Ivey, and
Karen B. Zur, *Editors*

RECENT ISSUES

December 2018
Facial Palsy: Diagnostic and Therapeutic Management
Teresa M. O, Nate Jowett, and
Tessa A. Hadlock, *Editors*

October 2018
Nasal Airway Obstruction
Jennifer A. Villwock and Ronald B.
Kuppersmith, *Editors*

August 2018
Geriatric Otolaryngology
Natasha Mirza and Jennifer Y. Lee, *Editors*

ISSUES OF RELATED INTEREST

Oral and Maxillofacial Surgery Clinics May 2018 (Vol. 30, No. 2)
Anesthesia
David W. Todd and Robert C. Bosack, *Editors*
Available at: https://www.oralmaxsurgery.theclinics.com/

Foreword

Delivering Otolaryngologic Care Safely and Successfully

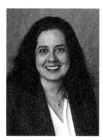

Sujana S. Chandrasekhar, MD, FACS, FAAOHNS
Consulting Editor

In 2000, when the Institute of Medicine published *To Err Is Human*,[1] the focus of the patient safety movement was on convincing both providers and patients that we had a safety problem. Currently, most people understand that patient safety is a real issue. Unfortunately, there are still an estimated 251,000 deaths[2] and over 1,000,000 nonfatal injuries[3] from medical errors annually in the United States. The focus now is on how to implement the best practices that we know exist. An additional challenge is creating a culture around safety, with leadership engagement. Physicians must be the change agents; without our strong commitment to patient safety, the needed improvements will not happen.

World Health Organization data show that nearly 43 million adverse events occur during the 421 million hospitalizations in the world every year, making patient harm the 14th leading worldwide cause of morbidity and mortality.[4] Of those adverse events, 83% could have been prevented, and 15% of health care spending is wasted dealing with all aspects of adverse events. Adverse patient safety outcomes include infections, surgical complications, inaccurate or delayed diagnoses, and unnecessary radiation exposure. Focused safety improvements result in both better patient outcomes and cost savings.

Dr Rahul Shah, the Guest Editor of this issue of *Otolaryngologic Clinics of North America* on Patient Safety, has led the charge within our subspecialty for years. His series of articles in the American Academy of Otolaryngology–Head and Neck Surgery *Bulletin* represents a treasure trove of information that many of us have relied on to improve our own practices. In this issue, Dr Shah has put together what I believe will be the definitive resource on patient safety in Otolaryngology for both individual physicians/practices and organizations.

In primary care, administrative errors account for 5% to 50% of all errors, indicating problems with systems and processes of delivering care. Otolaryngologists do much

Otolaryngol Clin N Am 52 (2019) xv–xvii
https://doi.org/10.1016/j.otc.2018.09.002
0030-6665/19/© 2018 Published by Elsevier Inc.

of their work outside of the intensive care/hospitalized patient arena, and systems science can have a major impact on their outcomes.

Physicians must lead the way, not only in practices and institutions but also in communities and nations. Even though we have known to wash our hands since Dr Lister's publication in March 1867,[5] health care–associated infections currently affect 7% to 10% of all hospitalized patients. Just using appropriate hand hygiene would reduce that by more than 50%. Patients can be willing partners with us as we move forward in the Safety arena. Being cognizant of our own implicit biases makes us better physicians in this, and all, patient care. I was particularly impressed by the articles "Rethinking Morbidity and Mortality Conference" and "Resident and Fellow Engagement in Safety and Quality." This is where current leaders engage future leaders, to better the health of society.

Much of what we do in Otolaryngology happens in the outpatient office setting, be it examination with reusable equipment, single-use tools, devices, audiometric testing, or office-based procedures. The articles on these subjects set an evidence-based framework for maximizing patient safety in each of these scenarios while avoiding unnecessary steps. Working as teams in the operating room or on the wards, Otolaryngologists can lead in patient safety through communication, be it in avoiding OR fires or dealing with a tough airway. Simulation, addressed here and in the entire October 2017 issue of *Otolaryngologic Clinics of North America* (Vol. 50, issue 5), can, indeed, save the day. Using public data for the bigger picture allows us to identify needs and create usable clinical indices for a targeted problem.

An iconic picture taken in 1932 shows 11 men on their lunch break (**Fig. 1**). They were construction workers building New York's Rockefeller Center,[6] and they are

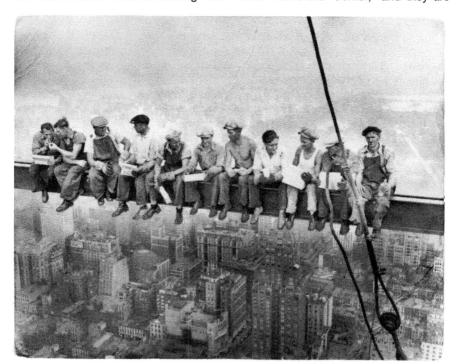

Fig. 1. Construction workers during the building of New York City's Rockefeller Center. (*From* Wikimedia Commons. Available at: https://commons.wikimedia.org/wiki/File:Lunch_atop_a_Skyscraper.jpg. Accessed September 11, 2018.)

just hanging out on this beam 850 feet above the sidewalk. There is nary a harness nor a hardhat in sight; one fellow is leaning forward, lighting up a cigarette, and one is drinking from an open bottle of alcohol. As an otologist, I will also point out that none are wearing ear protection. This could be the poster for nonsafety. Physicians have worked with society leaders to implement all sorts of patient safety and injury-prevention protocols; the article "Button Battery Safety: Industry and Academic Partnerships to Drive Change" highlights the possibilities of success with cross-discipline communication.

I learned a great deal about Patient Safety measures reading this issue of *Otolaryngologic Clinics of North America*. I commend Dr Shah on his leadership in this field and in collating this excellent collection of articles. I hope you enjoy it as well.

Sujana S. Chandrasekhar, MD, FACS, FAAOHNS
ENT & Allergy Associates, LLP
18 East 48th Street, 2nd Floor
New York, NY 10017, USA

Zucker School of Medicine at Hofstra-Northwell
Hempstead, NY 11549, USA

Icahn School of Medicine at Mount Sinai
New York, NY 10029, USA

E-mail address:
ssc@nyotology.com

REFERENCES

1. Institute of Medicine, Committee on Quality of Health Care in America. In: Kohn LT, Corrigan JM, Donaldson MS, editors. To err is human: building a safer health system. Washington, DC: The National Academies Press; 2000.
2. Makary MA, Daniel M. Medical error—the third leading cause of death in the US. BMJ 2016;353:i2139.
3. Weingart SN, Wilson RM, Gibberd RW, et al. Epidemiology of medical error. BMJ 2000;320(7237):774–7.
4. Available at: http://www.who.int/features/factfiles/patient_safety/en/. Accessed September 11, 2018.
5. Lister BJ. The classic: on the antiseptic principle in the practice of surgery. 1867. Clin Orthop Relat Res 2010;468(8):2012–6.
6. Available at: https://www.nytimes.com/2012/11/11/movies/lunch-atop-a-skyscraper-uncovered.html. Accessed September 11, 2018.

Preface

Patient Safety and Quality Improvement: Driving to New Frontiers

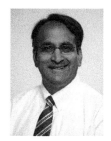

Rahul K. Shah, MD, MBA
Editor

Patient safety and quality improvement in health care, and specifically, in surgical specialties, is at a crossroads; the last decade has seen a myriad of initiatives resulting in order of magnitude improvements. The next decade will be challenging. Providers, hospitals, and organizations will need to "think differently" to drive toward zero harm.

This issue of *Otolaryngology Clinics of North America* is an attempt to start us on this journey of approaching quality and safety in the next decade with a different lens. Zero harm embodies the concept that patient safety and quality improvement is a journey of continuous improvement by elimination of iatrogenic harm from health care. This issue of *Otolaryngology Clinics of North America*, focusing on patient safety and quality improvement, looks backwards so that we can understand what we have learned; most of the content is aspirational and innovative, geared toward efforts to push our specialty toward zero harm. We begin the issue with a series of primers on important fundamentals of safety and quality. The subsequent articles attempt to provide a foundational description of work that has been accomplished and then tries to push our specialty to adopt novel approaches and techniques to move to zero harm. This will encompass a need to apply sophisticated leadership methods, embrace patient experience, and apply sophisticated publicly available data sets. Collaboratives and simulation are two areas that have been well known to result in marked improvements in safety and quality, and their application in Otolaryngology is burgeoning; the keys may lie with broader application of these areas. It will be imperative to avoid cognitive biases when approaching patient care with the paradigm of zero harm.

We have come to realize the crucial role of residents in being the face of the future. Indeed, data demonstrate that most residents practice in the manner that they are trained. Shouldn't we then consider how we incorporate trainees into our efforts to

Otolaryngol Clin N Am 52 (2019) xix–xx
https://doi.org/10.1016/j.otc.2018.09.001
0030-6665/19/© 2018 Published by Elsevier Inc.

drive high reliability? We highlight three areas that are desperate for attention in the modern patient safety and quality improvement movement: devices, ambulatory practices, and audiology. These three areas are the bedrock of Otolaryngology, yet remain relatively uncharted territory for safety and quality interventions.

We sincerely hope you find the contributions of these esteemed colleagues valuable when you consider how to help move your practice, department, or hospital to higher reliability and toward zero harm.

Rahul K. Shah, MD, MBA
Children's National Medical Center
George Washington University School
of Medicine & Health Sciences
West Wing, 5th Floor, Suite 403
111 Michigan Avenue, NW
Washington, DC 20010, USA

E-mail address:
rshah@childrensnational.org

Systems Science
A Primer on High Reliability

David W. Roberson, MD, MBA, FRCS[a],*, Elliana R. Kirsh, BM, BS[b]

KEYWORDS

- Systems • High reliability • Safety • Quality

KEY POINTS

- In the 21st century, most medical care is not delivered by a single physician but by a team.
- A team is a type of system, a set of people and things interacting together for a defined aim.
- The discipline of systems science concerns itself with how complex teams and organizations function.
- Systems science has had a major positive impact on safety and quality in such diverse disciplines as auto manufacturing, airline safety, and nuclear power generation.
- A modest understanding of how systems science applies to medical care can help improve safety and quality of care.

Only an ostrich could be unaware of the explosion of research and improvement efforts around quality and safety in the medical workplace and medical literature in the 18 years since the seminal report on the adverse consequences of medical errors in American medicine.[1,2] Nonetheless, many of us still struggle to grasp what quality means. After all, if we are well-trained and take good care of our patients, isn that not what quality means?

INDIVIDUAL EXCELLENCE IS NOT ENOUGH

In the 21st century, most medical care is not delivered by a single physician, but rather by a team. Patients entering the hospital for a simple procedure receive care from dozens or more providers. Teams can be more than the sum of their parts or less than the sum of their parts. If team members have well-defined and appropriate roles and work and communicate well together, good care will result. Likewise, if team members have poorly defined roles, do not work well together, and are not on the

Disclosure Statement: None.
a The Global Tracheostomy Collaborative, 165 Russett Road, West Roxbury, MA 02132, USA;
b Harvard Medical School, 1151 Beacon Street, Suite C1, Brookline, MA 02446, USA
* Corresponding author.
E-mail address: davidwroberson@me.com

Otolaryngol Clin N Am 52 (2019) 1–9
https://doi.org/10.1016/j.otc.2018.08.001
oto.theclinics.com

same page, good care is unlikely, even if each individual team member is supremely talented.

THE 21ST-CENTURY SURGEON IS THE LEADER OF A HIGH-PERFORMANCE TEAM

Team leadership comes with responsibility. If the surgeon knows that her team is dysfunctional, she has an obligation to her patients to do what she can to improve things. A surgeon who settles for being personally competent while accepting team dysfunction puts her patient as risk as surely as if she were to perform an operation that she is not trained for.

A TEAM IS A SYSTEM

Although systems can be incredibly complicated, we need not make the *concept* of systems complicated. A system is simply any set of people and things interacting together for a defined aim.[3] All of us have been working in complex systems our entire careers. Therefore, we have already learned many lessons about how systems work well (or do not). Still, a basic theoretical understanding of how systems work can improve our insights. The discipline of systems science concerns itself with how complex systems, teams, and organizations work. A great deal of high-quality research has been published in this domain, including data about how teams of people work well together.[2,4]

The application of systems science has had a major positive impact on safety and quality in such diverse disciplines as auto manufacturing, airline safety, and nuclear power generation. A modest understanding of how systems science applies to medical care can help us greatly in understanding why some teams perform well and others do not. When we grasp the role of systems science, we will come to see that quality as a discipline within medicine is, for the most part, concerned with improving team and system performance.

WHAT DETERMINES SYSTEM AND TEAM PERFORMANCE?

A system consists of elements that interact with each other. System performance is determined by both the quality of the system elements and the quality of their interactions. Just as no watchmaker can create a great watch from a set of bent and damaged parts, no system can perform well without high-quality elements. But the world's best set of watch parts will not magically assemble itself into a high-quality timepiece. How the parts are assembled is as important as how good the parts are.

The elements of a system can be people or things. In the case of a patient in the intensive care unit, the system elements may include dozens of physicians, midlevel providers, nurses, respiratory therapists, and other caregivers. The nonhuman parts include things such as the ventilator, the pulse oximeter, the infusion pump, the monitors, and the electronic medical record. If the people (eg, physicians or nurses) are not competent or the nonhuman elements are poor quality, the system will not perform at a high level.

However, high-quality elements alone do not guarantee good system function. A patient monitor, and its alarm system, may be perfectly designed and function perfectly. But if there are so many alarms that one is sounding every 3 minutes, the patient is at risk. They are at risk not because of equipment that is, dysfunctional per se, but because of dysfunctional system assembly without attention to the frequency and type of human–machine interactions.

This article first discusses the issues of system elements (people and things) and then discusses the importance of system interactions. It focuses primarily on human interactions, because these interactions typically matter the most and that are most amenable to change. Finally, this article reviews the concept of high reliability organizations (HROs), organizations that have a miniscule failure rate, and discuss whether it is realistic for a hospital or other health care system to become an HRO.

SYSTEM ELEMENTS

In modern American hospitals, rarely does improving quality mean that physician performance needs improvement. Most American physicians are well-trained, are committed, and perform at high levels as physicians. Improving quality also does not, in general, mean improving the performance of nonphysicians—nurses, physical therapists, physician assistants, scheduling assistants, and others. Physicians sometimes would prefer to believe that problems are due to others' performance issues. Most hospitals and offices are staffed with individuals who are completely capable of being part of a high performance team. Shortcomings, when they exist, are usually because individually competent individuals do not know how to interact and function as a team.

To the extent that individuals have performance issues, it should be noted that most individuals have a wide range of potential performance. On aircraft carriers, the failure rate for an incredibly complex task is miniscule. Many of the team members that make this possible are very young and might not be, on first blush, considered potential high reliability employees. But when these individuals join the navy, they go through a rigorous training and morale-building process. They are then surrounded by colleagues who expect and deliver high performance. With appropriate training, and support, individuals can markedly exceed what might be expected of them.[5] We should not immediately assume that the quality of a human being is fixed. Figuring out how to obtain better performance from current staff may often be a better strategy than replacing them.

What seems to be an individual performance problem may actually be a system failure, specifically, a failure of leadership. Team members who are not given clear expectations and good feedback and who are not treated as professional colleagues cannot perform at a high level, no matter how talented they may be.

System elements also include many things that the individual surgeon cannot control—the electronic medical record selected by the hospital, the organization of the operating room suite, or the brand of surgical equipment selected. Because these elements are beyond the influence of most readers, this article does not dwell on them.

System Interactions

System failure is more often due to poor quality interactions than with poor quality system elements. What does system science have to say on the subject of improving interactions, particularly human-to-human interactions? Several salient points are reviewed:

1. The importance of interactions;
2. Human error;
3. Respect for persons;
4. Common aims;
5. Leadership;
6. Unpredictability and emergence;
7. Local properties;

8. Measurement and feedback;
9. Cycle time; and
10. Standardization and customization.

Interactions Are More Numerous than Elements

As the number of team members increases linearly, the number of interactions increases disproportionately to the number of elements. In many systems, therefore, the quality of interactions is more important than the quality of the system elements. In 1 example, a large study showed that 30% of settled malpractice claims involved a communication failure.[6]

Human Error Is Ubiquitous

Although most health care providers perform at a high level, this factor does not imply that their performance is error free. Human errors are ubiquitous.[7–9] The Department of Defense estimates that that 80% to 90% of all failures are due to human error.[10] A study of commercial airline flight documented an average of 2 threats and 2 errors per flight.[11] However, cockpit errors almost never lead to crashes, because the aviation industry accepts the reality of human error and plans for it.[7] One of the most important techniques for managing human error is redundancy. Except in emergencies, life or death decisions should never be made by a 1 individual without backup. HROs ensure that backup is present for critical decisions. There processes are standardized, such as checklists, to ensure that important items are checked. HROs also go to great lengths to ensure that those responsible for double-checking decisions are free to speak up. If a copilot (or a nurse) is afraid to raise a concern, the pilot (or the surgeon) will have no safety net when he makes mistakes.[7,9]

Respect for Persons

Failure to treat others with respect poisons a team in multiple ways. If individuals are not treated with respect, they do not perform well. Team members who are afraid to speak up cannot perform their backup function for critical decisions. Unhappy people interact poorly—and poor quality interactions degrade team performance. Just as putting a sand grain at a single point in a watch may not seriously damage its function, a single bad interaction may not greatly threaten care. But if large numbers of human-to-human interactions are indifferent, unpleasant, or disrespectful, the care system is like a watch with a sand grain stuck in every cog.

Many organizations are currently attempting to improve human interactions and empower workers by creating and maintaining a just culture.[12] In such a culture, all members are equally empowered to speak up and to contribute to organizational improvement without fear of negative response.

Common Aims

Many priorities compete with each other during patient care. The resident may want to be taught the simpler elements of the case. The fellow may want to have an opportunity to perform the more difficult parts. The attending may want to get to her clinic by 2:00 PM. The nurse may be focused on ensuring that protocols are followed and instruments are handled safely. But if it is impossible to achieve all these goals in the available time and there is not an open discussion of how to compromise around these goals, it is likely that everyone will leave frustrated. Team members cannot work well together if there is not a clear understanding of their shared goals.

Likewise, institutional mission and values statements can be very valuable if genuine. If a mission statement genuinely reflects the organization's values, and decisions consistently conform to the stated mission, and this process can be unifying and morale building. Conversely, if institutional leadership frequently makes decisions that are not consistent with the mission statement, staff will quickly see this for the charade it is.

Leadership

Leadership is of great importance in high performing human systems, but not in the way that one might expect. Quality is a local characteristic—the quality of patient care is determined entirely by what front-line doctors, nurses, and other providers do. Leadership's role is, therefore, not to prescribe behaviors to front-line workers, but to empower them.[13] If individual physicians, nurses, and other providers are empowered to address system problems, to call out troublesome issues, and to contribute to solutions, they will make local positive changes. Conversely, if all decisions are made in a top-down fashion and if those who point out problems are ignored or blamed, system performance will suffer. Likewise, the critical task for the surgeon team leader is not to make every decision, but to empower and support his colleagues and team members.

Unpredictability

All large systems behave unpredictably.[4] A new policy may make perfect sense in the cardiology department, but when deployed to other departments may have negative unintended consequences. Moreover, large systems manifest "emergence"—the systems manifest behavior that would be difficult if not impossible to predict, particularly after significant changes.

Systems Are Local and Unique

A policy or procedure that works incredibly well in one hospital or department may fail in another. Because of the phenomena of unpredictability and uniqueness, all system changes should be approached carefully. There are some activities that will almost always improve a system (eg, improving interpersonal interactions, shortening cycle time). Solutions to specific problems, however, may work well in one system and not in another. It is simply not possible to predict every outcome in complex systems.[4] System solutions should not be directly imported from another hospital or department without some careful thought about how they will perform locally. Any significant change should be monitored carefully to understand all the outcomes of that change—not just the expected ones.

Measurement and Feedback

High-quality systems have multiple feedback loops. Measurement and feedback may be quite simple and still effective. If a nursing team changes their phone triage practices, the most effective feedback strategy is probably simply to ask them if it is working. Other measures need to be defined much more formally. If one wishes to compare outcomes for cardiac surgery between centers, elaborate risk stratification is necessary. However, some type of measurement and feedback is essential.[14–16]

In theory, the more measurement and feedback that is built into a system, the better it will perform. But in reality, measurement and feedback require resources and can take energy away from the core system functions. It is important, therefore to:

1. Measure enough things to know how you are doing.
2. Measure them well enough so the results are believable.
3. Not to allow the measurement burden to overwhelm system function.

Often it is important to work with good enough measures rather than to insist on perfection in measurement.

Cycle Time

Shortening cycle time is almost always a win. Finish and sign your notes today. If your team has a new recommendation, make sure the primary team knows about it now—do not wait for your resident to finish the note later tonight. Answer phone calls and pages promptly. Do not make the rest of the system wait on you.

Standardization and Customization

Standardization protocols and routine improve performance for tasks that must be done repeatedly. In the Global Tracheostomy Collaborative, hospitals are encouraged to develop standard clinical processes and pathways for all tracheostomy patients, which leads to a significant decrease in tracheostomy harm in diverse hospitals worldwide.[17–19] Practice guidelines can ensure that all patients receive a basic level of care and greatly reduce simple errors and oversights.[20]

Standardization is like the foundation of a house. Protocols and practice guidelines help us to build this foundation for every patient. But each patient needs customized care—which is the house we build on the foundation of standardization. In fact, by standardizing routine processes, more time can be devoted to customizing the patient's care.

High Reliability Organizations

The term HRO describes organizations with extremely low failure rates. Examples include naval aircraft carriers, commercial aviation, nuclear power plants, and some but not all manufacturing enterprises. The seminal work on HROs remains "Managing the Unexpected" by Weick and Sutcliffe.[21] Because HROs are all complex systems, there are parallels between principles of systems science and what is observed in HROs in the field. Weick and Sutcliffe noted 5 basic principles common to all of the HROs that they studied:

1. Preoccupation with failure,
2. Reluctance to simplify,
3. Sensitivity to operations,
4. Resilience, and
5. Deference to expertise.

Preoccupation with Failure

HROs treat every failure or near miss as a learning opportunity. They go to great lengths to create a blame-free culture so that as many problems as possible can be reported, analyzed, and serve as grist for iterative improvements.[22,23]

Reluctance to Simplify

HROs do not try to impose simple, one-size-fits-all, top-down policies or solutions. Instead, they take the effort to understand the various components of the enterprise and to learn the gritty details about how things work. They recognize that system improvement is an iterative, small-scale activity and that it depends on really understanding the details.

Sensitivity to Operations

If things are going better or worse recently, HROs want to know why. If 1 department or area is struggling, or there is a new pattern of activity, they want to investigate and understand it. Again, they go to great lengths to create an open culture so that front-line workers and midlevel managers are encouraged to share operational issues with leadership.

Resilience

HROs recognize that human error is ubiquitous and that complex systems can also fail. Therefore, they spend time thinking in advance about what types of failures to expect and build plans and capacity to manage problems. They build rescue procedures such that, when a failure occurs, it can be identified and rectified before it causes a catastrophe.

Deference to Expertise

HRO leadership does not try to solve problems. Rather, leadership identifies the experts within the organization and listens to them. The front-line workers and front-line managers are the first ones called in an emergency. Top-down decision making is anathema to HROs.

Weick and Sutcliffe[21] summarize the 5 principles they have outlined as "organizational mindfulness." The organization and the people in it do not simply do their job for a period of time. The organization (through its human members) is doing the day's work, but also constantly taking time to reflect, to notice how things are going, and to look out for themes or areas that need attention. Thus, the organization will notice system problems early and has the opportunity to attend to them early on.

Can Hospitals Become High Reliability Organizations?

No hospital even approaches the miniscule failure rate that HROs achieve. In fairness, providing medical care to multiple critically ill patients is in many ways are more complex than (for example) commercial aviation.

Hospitals can make major specific improvements by following the principles of system science—for example, there have been great strides in reducing central line infections,[24] improving handoffs,[25] and tracheostomy outcomes.[17–19] However, it is not yet clear that a hospital can truly become a top-to-bottom HRO, with miniscule failure rates in all of its operations. Moreover, it is not clear what the path from the current state to HRO would be[26,27]—what steps to take and in what order—because no hospital has yet accomplished this goal,[28,29] although a number of institutions are making sustained efforts toward total reliability.[30–32] For the moment, whether hospitals can ever become HROs and the correct path to that goal remains uncertain and awaits much additional research and implementation efforts.[24,33]

SUMMARY

Medical care in the 21st-century is delivered within a complex system. Being an excellent surgeon no longer is enough; the surgeon must take the responsibility for leading a high performance team. A basic understanding of complex systems, HROs, and QI processes will make the 21st-century surgery far more competent in her role as team leader.

REFERENCES

1. Kohn L, Corrigan J, Donaldson M. To err is human: building a safer health system. Washington, DC: National Academy Press; 2000.
2. Manser T. Teamwork and patient safety in dynamic domains of healthcare: a review of the literature. Acta Anaesthesiol Scand 2009;53(2):143–51.
3. Nolan T. Understanding medical systems. Annals of Internal Medicine 1999;128: 293–8.
4. Bar-Yam Y. Dynamics of complex systems. Reading (MA): Perseus Books; 1997.
5. Hutchins E. Cognition in the wild. Boston: MIT Press; 1995.
6. CRICO Strategies. Malpractice risk in communication failures; annual benchmarking report. Boston: The Risk Management Foundation of the Harvard Medical Institutions, Inc.; 2015 (registration required for download).
7. Helmreich RL. On error management: lessons from aviation. BMJ 2000;320: 781–5.
8. Perrow. Normal accidents. New York: Basic Books; 1984.
9. Reason J. Human error. Cambridge (England): Cambridge University Press; 1990.
10. US Department of Defense. 2005 Department of defense human factors analysis and classification system: a mishap investigation and data analysis tool. 2005. Available at: http://www.uscg.mil/safety/docs/pdf/hfacs.pdf. Accessed August 2, 2018.
11. Klinect JR, Wilhelm JA, Helmreich RL. Proceedings of the tenth international symposium on aviation psychology. Threat and error management: data from line operations safety audits. Columbus (OH): Ohio State University; 1999. p. 683–8.
12. Frankel AS, Leonard MW, Denham CR. Fair and just culture, team behavior, and leadership engagement: the tools to achieve high reliability. Health Serv Res 2006;41(4p2):1690–709.
13. Reinertsen JL. Physicians as leaders in the improvement of healthcare systems. Ann Intern Med 1998;128:833–8.
14. Montroy J, Breau RH, Cnossen S, et al. Change in adverse events after enrollment in the National Surgical Quality Improvement Program: a systematic review and meta-analysis. PLoS One 2016;11(1):e0146254.
15. Shah RK, Stey AM, Jatana KR, et al. Identification of opportunities for quality improvement and outcome measurement in pediatric otolaryngology. JAMA Otolaryngol Head Neck Surg 2014;140(11):1019–26.
16. Shah RK, Welborn L, Ashktorab S, et al. Safety and outcomes of outpatient pediatric otolaryngology procedures at an ambulatory surgery center. Laryngoscope 2008;118(11):1937–40.
17. Cameron TS, McKinstry A, Burt SK, et al. Outcomes of patients with spinal cord injury before and after introduction of an interdisciplinary tracheostomy team. Crit Care Resusc 2009;11(1):14–9.
18. Hettige R, Arora A, Ifeacho S, et al. Improving tracheostomy management through design, implementation and prospective audit of a care bundle: how we do it. Clin Otolaryngol 2008;33(5):488–91.
19. McGrath BA, Lynch J, Bonvento B, et al. Evaluating the quality improvement impact of the Global Tracheostomy Collaborative in four diverse NHS hospitals. BMJ Qual Improv Rep 2017;6(1) [pii:bmjqir.u220636.w7996].
20. Collins SJ, Newhouse R, Porter J, et al. Effectiveness of the surgical safety checklist in correcting errors: a literature review applying Reason's Swiss cheese model. AORN J 2014;100(1):65–79.

21. Karl E, Weick KE, Sutcliffe KM. Managing the unexpected: sustained performance in a complex world. 3rd edition. Hoboken (NJ): Wiley; 2015.
22. Ferroli P, Caldiroli D, Acerbi F, et al. Application of an aviation model of incident reporting and investigation to the neurosurgical scenario: method and preliminary data. Neurosurg Focus 2012;33(5):E7.
23. Van Spall H, Kassam A, Tollefson TT. Near-misses are an opportunity to improve patient safety: adapting strategies of high reliability organizations to healthcare. Curr Opin Otolaryngol Head Neck Surg 2015;23(4):292–6.
24. Shabot MM, Monroe D, Inurria J, et al. Memorial Hermann: high reliability from board to bedside. Jt Comm J Qual Patient Saf 2013;39(6):AP1–5.
25. Dingley C, Daugherty K, Derieg MK, et al. Improving patient safety through provider communication strategy enhancements. In: Henriksen K, Battles JB, Keyes MA, et al, editors. Advances in patient safety: new directions and alternative approaches (Vol. 3: performance and tools). Rockville (MD): Agency for Healthcare Research and Quality; 2008.
26. Alexander JA, Hearld LR. The science of quality improvement implementation. Developing capacity to make a difference. Med Care 2011;49:S6–20.
27. Dixon NM, Shofer M. Struggling to invent high-reliability organizations in health care settings: insights from the field. Health Serv Res 2006;41(4p2):1618–32.
28. Chassin MR, Loeb JM. The ongoing quality improvement journey: next stop, high reliability. Health Aff 2011;30(4):559–68.
29. Chassin MR, Loeb JM. High-reliability health care: getting there from here. Milbank Q 2013;91(3):459–90.
30. Pronovost PJ, Armstrong CM, Demski R, et al. Creating a high-reliability health care system: improving performance on core processes of care at Johns Hopkins Medicine. Acad Med 2015;90(2):165–72.
31. Pronovost PJ, Holzmueller CG, Callender T, et al. Sustaining reliability on accountability measures at the Johns Hopkins Hospital. Jt Comm J Qual Patient Saf 2016;42(2):51–60.
32. Rosen M, Mueller BU, Milstone AM, et al. Creating a pediatric joint council to promote patient safety and quality, governance, and accountability across Johns Hopkins Medicine. Jt Comm J Qual Patient Saf 2017;43(5):224–31.
33. Sullivan JL, Rivard PE, Shin MH, et al. Applying the high reliability health care maturity model to assess hospital performance: a VA case study. Jt Comm J Qual Patient Saf 2016;42(9):389–99.

Leadership Driving Safety and Quality

Erin L. McKean, MD, MBA[a,b,*], Carl H. Snyderman, MD, MBA[c,d]

KEYWORDS

- Quality • Safety • Leadership • Systems-based practice • Value

KEY POINTS

- Technological advances are leveling the hierarchy of health care, leading to more collaborative, innovative problem solving.
- Flexible, skilled leaders are required at all levels in the health care system.
- Leadership includes envisioning the direction of the group, strategically planning activities toward the vision, executing the strategic plan by assuring alignment of activities with goals, reflecting on progress and failures, and course correction (plan revision).
- Management implies a formal position of supervisory capacity with expressly denoted goals, roles, and expectations.
- Different leadership models may be best used in these different leadership and management roles.

INTRODUCTION

Most safety and quality efforts fail not due to lack of metrics, data, or proposed solutions but rather due to failure in execution of change management. Could executive-level leadership and organizational culture have an impact? Could a relative lack of frontline quality and safety leadership be at fault? Health care culture is traditionally hierarchical, and medical providers have long placed value on autonomy in practice and problem solving. Team-based, motivational leadership training has not been emphasized throughout most of medical training, and, until recently, systems-based practice was a topic for academics, not necessarily a conversation piece for those

The authors have nothing to disclose.

[a] Otolaryngology–Head and Neck Surgery, University of Michigan, 1904 Taubman Center, 1500 East Medical Center Drive, Ann Arbor, MI 48109, USA; [b] Neurosurgery, University of Michigan, 1904 Taubman Center, 1500 East Medical Center Drive, Ann Arbor, MI 48109, USA; [c] Department of Otolaryngology, University of Pittsburgh School of Medicine, The Eye & Ear Institute, 200 Lothrop Street, Suite 500, Pittsburgh PA 15213, USA; [d] Department of Neurological Surgery, University of Pittsburgh School of Medicine, The Eye & Ear Institute, 200 Lothrop Street, Suite 500, Pittsburgh PA 15213, USA

* Corresponding author. Otolaryngology–Head and Neck Surgery, University of Michigan, 1904 Taubman Center, 1500 East Medical Center Drive, Ann Arbor, MI 48109.

E-mail address: elmk@med.umich.edu

Otolaryngol Clin N Am 52 (2019) 11–22
https://doi.org/10.1016/j.otc.2018.08.002
0030-6665/19/© 2018 Elsevier Inc. All rights reserved.

at the front lines of care delivery. Transformative forces, such as changing payment models and information technology, are demanding a leveling of the hierarchy and growth in collaborative, innovative problem solving. Flexible, skilled leaders are required at all levels in the health care system.

Who are these health care leaders? When speaking of safety and quality, any participant in the value chain (eg, the care of the patient, directly or indirectly) may lead. There are leaders in formal positions of authority and those empowered individuals who lead change in daily activities. In this article, manager and leader are used almost synonymously, although there is a conceptual distinction between the two. Leadership in simplest terms implies directing a group or organization. In a more expanded definition, leadership includes envisioning the direction of the group, strategically planning activities toward the vision, executing the strategic plan by assuring alignment of activities with goals, reflecting on progress and failures, and course correction (plan revision). Management, on the other hand, implies a formal position of supervisory capacity with expressly denoted goals, roles, and expectations. Different leadership models may be best used in these different leadership and management roles.

Regardless of formal position, all participants in quality and safety efforts need to have certain attributes, behaviors, and skills to successfully lead change. Dedicated leadership training has been shown to be vital for transforming systems of care and engaging all members of a health care team. Multiple institutions now encourage leadership training for all levels of employees, and several organizations are exemplars of great strides in safety and quality that have been achieved through system-wide leadership training and empowerment (thereby changing culture and demonstrating commitment to these important efforts).

EVIDENCE FOR THE ROLE OF LEADERSHIP IN SAFETY AND QUALITY OUTCOMES

Industrial studies have long shown the importance of organizational culture (or climate) in creating and sustaining meaningful safety outcomes.[1,2] Safety communication (between workers and managers) and leadership's declared commitment to safety give cues to workers regarding the importance of safety as well as the need for prioritization of safety measures.[3] Groups with high levels of safety communication and a declared commitment to safety showed lower levels of worker injury in manufacturing. Consistent action regarding safety and quality is critical in creating culture.

In addition, participative management, in which workers are involved in decision-making processes has been shown to be a better predictor of safety outcomes than authoritative management.[4] This management style involves communication, involvement, and empowerment in a setting of relationships characterized by trust, openness, and honesty. Participative management focuses less on individual blame (which is convenient though ineffective in preventing future problems) and more on analysis of root causes of problems.

Participative management, linked to transformational leadership style (discussed later), has also been shown to be vital in creating a culture of safety in health care. In 2010, Vogus and colleagues[5] reviewed industrial safety, specifically health care literature, proposing a participative culture model of "enabling, enacting and elaborating." *Enabling* requires leaders to draw attention to safety within the organization and also to empower frontline workers to act deliberately when caring for patients. *Enacting* means having systems to act on safety concerns expressed by enabled workers as well as mobilizing resources to create safety systems and achieve goals. *Elaborating* focuses on the plan-do-study-act (PDSA) process (which has been found highly valuable in quality improvement collaboratives),[6] taking learning and processes from a small-scale to larger-scale system-wide practices, while continually learning and refining.

McKinsey also looked at more direct frontline managers and leaders, developing a "clinical operations excellence" approach to motivate those at the forefront of care and achieve transformative goals.[7] Broome and colleagues noted the critical aspect of communicating improved patient outcomes, rather than focusing on cost control or other secondary metrics that go more to the bottom line. They found that leaders often fail to recognize the importance of frontline capability-building and resource mobilization. They additionally found, consistent with other studies, that to achieve strong results in terms of quality and safety, all leaders at all levels must be engaged and must champion and role model the behavior they want to see. McKinsey & Company's London office crafted an earlier white paper that spoke to distributed leadership, identifying 3 archetypes of clinical leaders: institutional leaders, service leaders, and frontline leaders.[8] This study emphasized the specific development of these leaders and again noted the ability of clinician leaders to be influential champions, deeply committed to high-performance.

As a side note, there is evidence that safety climate may vary within units of an organization.[9] Similar results have been found in the health care setting, and there is additional information to show that frontline workers' perception of safety are more aligned with actual outcomes than those of senior managers.[10] These studies reinforce the need for aligned leadership and activities throughout an organization, both at the executive level and at the frontlines of care, in multiple departments and divisions. Direct supervisors and vocal followers can have great sway in the success or failure of institutional efforts.

Structurally, leadership performance can be shaped by careful vetting and alignment of incentives. The Agency for Healthcare Research and Quality (AHRQ) reviewed the role of hospital managers in quality and safety in 2014, finding significant positive associations with quality to include compensation attached to quality, using quality improvement measures, and having a hospital board quality committee.[11]

In terms of executive leadership, in 2013 an AHRQ study summarized the role of hospital boards in oversight of quality and patient safety.[12] Hospital boards traditionally consist of community leaders who may have little background in health care quality and patient safety, but the role of the board is essential in fostering safety practices. Overall, high-performing hospitals were found to have skilled board members and standardized processes for prioritizing safety and quality. This is consistent with the data from industry, discussed previously, confirming the need for consistent communication and declared commitment to safety and quality efforts.

As a final note, safety and quality are not interchangeable concepts, and evidence shows that different tools and processes are necessary in achieving each. Nonetheless, concurrent implementation of quality and safety initiatives results in greater combined benefits.[13] Adept leaders must understand the culture necessary as well as relevant tools and metrics to achieve safety and quality goals alike.

HEALTH CARE LEADERSHIP MODELS

Although it is apparent from the evidence that leadership is essential in creating culture, producing highly effective clinician leaders in health care has often faltered. Medical training has traditionally rewarded independence and competitiveness over team-based problem-solving.[14] Moreover, the system may actually disincentivize effective clinicians from taking leadership roles.[8] Leadership development requires understanding leadership models applicable to health care and a continual maturation of specific competencies.

Multiple models of leadership exist, and these are helpful in understanding leadership fit for the purpose of developing quality and safety programs. **Table 1** shows a sampling of published leadership models. This sampling is not all-inclusive and does not incorporate the previously described management models of Vogus and colleagues ("enabling, enacting, elaborating")[5] or McKinsey & Company ("clinical operations excellence").[7]

Although not specific to health care, one of the oldest leadership frameworks in the study of organizational behavior is Burns'[15] and then Bass and Avolio's[16] theory of full-range (transformational, transactional and laissez-faire) leadership. Transformational leadership focuses on trusting, individualized relationships aimed at exceeding goals whereas transactional leadership focuses on explicit expectations with explicit rewards or roles. Transformational leaders tend to be inspirational, with the ability to enact great change within an organization. Quinn[17] described the "fundamental state of leadership" for transformational leaders by the attributes of being results-centered, internally directed, other-focused, and externally open. Transactional leaders tend to be less charismatic, relying more on rules, policies, and procedures along with conditional rewards. Finally, laissez-faire leaders are generally disconnected nonleaders. Spinelli[18] studied the transformation-transactional-laissez faire model in hospital administration, finding that health care administrative leaders possess both transformational and transactional leadership styles. The more transformational the leader, the more likely a direct report was to exert additional effort, express satisfaction, and find the leader to be more effective.

Value-based interactions between leaders and subordinates encompass openness, trust, and loyalty and are characteristic of transformational leadership,[26] and transformational leaders tend to encourage a participative leadership structure, empowering those at the front lines. These same attributes have been found to be critical in introduction of new technology in the operating room.[27] Communication of a motivating rationale and allowing open feedback from all team members regardless of status led to most effective implementation. Although this study did not directly address safety and quality, these are logical secondary outcomes.

Evidence has shown that transformational and transactional leadership styles are complementary.[1] Transformational behaviors create a climate in which safety and quality are valued, encourage free flow of information, and contribute to constructive problem solving rather than a blame culture. Transactional behaviors assure that regulatory and programmatic requirements are met and that resources are mobilized. This is important to understand and leverage specifically in the context of supervisors and middle managers. One style is not better than the other, and a different leadership approach may be needed to suit a particular task or role.

COMPETENCIES OF LEADERS

To build mindful leaders who can apply leadership theory to the actual task at hand, organizations should consider the competencies required for leading teams and organizations. To build culture and meet an organization's quality and safety needs, leaders must have fundamental attributes, behaviors, and skills. In a Becker Hospital review online post, 9 essential leadership skills were cited.[28] These are setting a vision, communicating strategically, creating an environment of constructive accountability and constructive conflict, removing barriers to success (ie, allocation of resources), coaching, celebrating success, earning trust, self-awareness, and collaboration. At

Table 1
Sampling of published leadership models

Model	Developer(s)	Principles Applied to Safety and Quality Leadership
Transformational, Transactional, and Laissez-Faire Leadership; Fundamental State of Leadership	Burns,[15] 1979; Bass & Avolio,[16] 1995; Spinelli,[18] 2006; Quinn,[19] 2005	Importance of personal and team values; motivating others; visioning; active engagement of team in creating positive change
Competing Values Framework	Cameron et al,[20] 2006	Values-based motivation and innovation in problem-solving; respect for diversity
National Center for Healthcare Leadership Competency Model	National Center for Healthcare Leadership,[21] 2006	Application of individual leadership attributes to solving systems-based problems in teams; focus on influence, strategy and execution of change processes
Medical Leadership Competency Framework, 3rd edition	National Health Service Institute for Innovation and Improvement and Academy of Medical Royal Colleges, UK,[22] 2011	Training-level-appropriate, staged development of leadership and management skills with a focus on shared leadership (and team-based problem solving)
A3 Lean Management Process	Toyota Production System, described by Shook in *Managing to Learn*,[23] 2008	Empowerment of health care team in systems-based problem solving, shared leadership; leadership communication behaviors
Functional Results-Oriented Health Care Leadership Model	Al-Touby,[24] 2012	Improved/exceptional patient outcomes at center of leadership and change in health care; results-oriented problem solving
The Healthcare Leadership Alliance Model	Stefl,[25] 2008	Emphasis on defining competencies to meet future professional leadership requirements; importance of management skills for the leader

the University of Michigan, leadership competencies have been determined to be core competencies for graduating medical students, and other institutions have concurrently been developing leadership milestones and competencies. In the book, *Health Systems Science*,[14] competencies of health care leaders are described (**Table 2**). These include

- Foundational leadership
  - Leadership in health care must be predicated on patient-centeredness and professionalism.
  - The American College of Physician Executives reviewed literature and data regarding performances of hospitals run by physicians versus nonclinicians, finding a competitive advantage for physician leaders because of "extensive

knowledge of the 'core business' of caring for human beings. They have learned, lived, and breathed patient care."[29]

- Self-management
  - In order to lead others, leaders should first lead themselves. This means developing one's own emotional intelligence and maintaining an achievement orientation.
  - Leaders must serve selflessly, placing the goals of the organization and the team ahead of personal accomplishment.
  - Leaders act as role models and their behavior has an impact on the safety climate.
  - There is evidence to support that effectively leading one's self is associated with effectively leading others.[30]
- Team management
  - Leaders must pay attention both to the taskwork (what is being done) and teamwork (how the work is being done).[31]
  - Leaders must develop relationships of trust and openness, being careful not to silence voices within the organization.[32]
  - Leaders must mentor and develop new talent.[33]
- Influence and communication
  - Leaders must communicate effectively, tailoring their messages to different audiences, styles, and venues. This includes written, visual, and face-to-face communication.
  - Leaders should be skilled advocates and be comfortable having challenging conversations.
  - Leaders must influence organizations, being able to navigate politics of an organization and system.
  - A 2016 national survey of physicians by athenaInsight found that only 20% of physicians feel engaged in their organization, but 2-way communication with influential leaders can build frontline engagement.[34] The management skill category most valued by physicians was communication.
- Systems-based practice
  - Leaders must have in-depth knowledge of the health care environment.
  - Business knowledge and skills are essential in effecting change.
  - The Accreditation Council for Graduate Medical Education and American Board of Medical Specialties have identified systems-based practice as 1 of 6 core competencies, thus requiring training and proficiency in the delivery of safe, high-quality care.[35]
- Executing toward a vision
  - Leaders must develop a vision as well as a strategy to work toward that end.
  - The great importance of creating a culture of safety and quality has already been emphasized. Again, leadership, formally and informally, is a critical driver of safety and quality outcomes.
  - Leaders use the PDSA model to create sustainable solutions.

LEADERSHIP DOMAINS AND SHARED LEADERSHIP

Leaders in the complex health care environment cannot possibly be experts in all aspects of health care and the business of delivering that care. Creating a broad team of expert leaders who are committed to safety and quality optimizes systemization of efforts. Consideration should be given to all portions of the value chain for patients, including

Table 2
Health care leadership competencies

Leadership Foundations	Self-Management	Team Management	Influence and Communication	Systems-Based Practice	Executing toward a Vision
• Maintaining patient centeredness • Professionalism	• Serving selflessly • Achievement orientation/pursuing excellence • Emotional intelligence	• Relationship management • Developing new talent • Human resources	• Communicating effectively • Advocacy • Having challenging conversations • Navigating politics	• Knowledge of the health care environment • Business knowledge and skills	• Vision and strategy • Creating culture • Creating sustainable solutions

From Grethlein SJ, Clyne B, McKean E. Leadership in health care. In: Skochelak SE, et al, editors. Health Systems Science. 1st edition. Philadelphia: Elsevier; 2017. p. 92–104; with permission.

- Patient logistics (inbound and outbound)
  - Referrals and scheduling
  - Coordination at discharge
- Operations
  - Day-to-day patient care (by all members of the health care team)
  - Quality and safety programs
- Communications
  - Messaging, written media
  - Web site
  - Community presence
- Information technology
  - Electronic health record interface for patients and clinicians
  - Information sharing
  - Information technology systems for other business functions
- Marketing
  - Patient satisfaction and needs assessment
- Finance
  - Allocation of scarce resources
  - Changing payment models' impact on care
  - Creation of incentive plans
- Accounting
  - Audit functions
  - Billing and collections
  - Payables
- Human resources
  - Hiring
  - Scheduling
  - Conflict resolution
- Legal
  - Compliance
  - Risk management
- Executive
  - Visioning
  - Strategy

CREATING A CULTURE OF TEAM LEADERSHIP, SAFETY, AND QUALITY: LEAN ENTERPRISES

As discussed previously, organizational culture is fundamental to achieving quality and safety outcomes. Lean thinking, a management style originally associated with the Toyota Production System, focuses on doing more with less. There is a focus on eliminating waste and leaving only the value-added steps in a process. More important than outcomes alone is a robust process called A3 thinking.[23] This process can be integrated into an entire organization and requires

- Mentored frontline engagement
- Coaches who are invested in building the problem-solving skills of the problem owner
- Detailed problem identification
- Deep understanding of processes
- Going to the *gemba* (actual place where value-added work occurs)

- Root cause analysis (including the practice of 5 Whys, or asking why repeatedly until the true root cause if found) and data analysis
- Proposal and structured evaluation of countermeasures to problems
- Plan-do-check-act

Senior leadership plays a major role in lean management. Lean consultant and organizational psychologist Dr David Mann[36] noted that "80% of the effort [in Lean transformations] is expended on changing leaders' practices and behaviors, and ultimately their mindset." Leadership lean tasks include supporting resources for cross-boundary collaboration, gemba walks (going to the front lines of care to see the work and discuss opportunities for improvement), collaboration in process management (measurement and accountability), teaching, and role modeling. Consistent senior leadership engagement in these tasks is key to producing a lasting culture of quality improvement and safety.

THE VALUE OF LEADERSHIP DRIVING SAFETY AND QUALITY

Several health care systems and alliances have been exemplars of leadership driving a culture of value.

- ThedaCare in Wisconsin began a cultural change in 1997, with leadership specifically focusing on a change culture and consistently (and visibly) pursuing quality improvement. They noted that "preparing your staff is the hardest part" and invested significant time, money, and resources to develop staff.[37]
  - In terms of diabetes care, the number of diabetic patients receiving a yearly eye examination rose from 65% to 85%, patients with hemoglobin A_{1c} levels below 8.0 rose from 43% to 60%, and the average hemoglobin A_{1c} levels decreased from 8.7 to 7.6.
  - System-wide turnover is at 9% compared with an industry average of 17%.
  - In 2004, they noted $3.3 million in savings and reduced accounts receivable from 56 days to 44 days (equating to $12 million in cash flow).[38]
  - Phone triage times decreased by 35%, reducing hold time from 89 seconds to 58 seconds.
  - Admission clinical paperwork time was reduced by 50%.
- Virginia Mason Medical Center in Washington began using lean management principles in 2002. They maintained a no-layoff policy, required employee attendance at an Introduction to Lean course and deeply changed the culture through the engagement of committed, inspiring senior leadership.[38]
  - They specifically found the need for leaders to be visible, vocal champions of lean management, creating a culture of innovation (with permission to fail and to set stretch goals) and a relentless pursuit of value (increased quality and reduced waste).
  - In 2004, inventory was down 53% from the start of lean management in 2002, and floor space had actually decreased with increased productivity.
  - By eliminating waste, significant capital expense plans were no longer necessary, saving approximately $8 million by cancellation of procedural and surgical suite expansions.
- Michigan Medicine has a quality department with a mission of providing safe, quality care for patient and families. There are 7 divisions, which include clinical design and innovation, clinical quality and training, Michigan Program on value Enhancement, patient safety, performance improvement, program management, and quality analytics.[39]

- Through the office of patient safety, a patient safety event team evaluates harm events, manages institutional response, and develops action plans. In 2017, more than 50 reviews were performed with the goal of creating a culture of safety.
- Through multidisciplinary teamwork facilitated by institutional leadership, a new partnership between emergency department and cardiology allows for patients to be treated in the emergency department for atrial fibrillation and sent home for management rather than admitted. In 1 year, 96 patients avoided admission, improving patient satisfaction and opening critically needed inpatient beds.

SUMMARY

Leaders in health care play a large role in successful achievement of quality and safety goals through an overt commitment to both quality and safety, fostering a culture of quality improvement and clear and consistent communication of goals and plans. Quality and safety tools and processes by themselves are limited; leaders create the environment where these processes thrive and propagate. Specific training for frontline providers, managers, and staff is critical in developing skilled leaders with a quality and safety orientation. Many models now exist for organizational leadership development, and exemplars of quality and safety leadership have openly shared the keys to their successes in order for others to raise the bar.

REFERENCES

1. Flin R, Yule S. Leadership for safety: industrial experience. Qual Saf Health Care 2004;13(Suppl II):ii45–51.
2. Hofmann D, Morgeson FP, Gerras SJ. Climate as a moderator of the relationship between leader-member exchange and content specific citizenship: safety climate as an exemplar. J Appl Psychol 2003;88(1):170–8.
3. Zohar D. The effects of leadership dimensions, safety climate, and assigned priorities on minor injuries in work groups. J Organ Behav 2002;23:75–92.
4. O'Dea A, Flin R. Site managers and safety leadership in the offshore oil and gas industry. Saf Sci 2001;37:39–57.
5. Vogus TJ, Sutcliffe KM, Weick KE. Doing no harm: enabling, enacting and elaborating a culture of safety in health care. Acad Manage Perspec 2010;24:60–77.
6. Nembhard IM. Learning and improving in quality improvement collaboratives: which collaborative features do participants value most? Health Serv Res 2009;44(2):359–78.
7. Broome B, Grote K, Scott J, et al. Clinical operations excellence: unlocking a hospital's true potential. McKinsey&Company white paper; 2013. Available at: https://healthcare.mckinsey.com/clinical-operations-excellence-unlocking-hospital%E2%80%99s-true-potential. Accessed January 1, 2015.
8. Mountford J, Webb C. Clinical leadership: unlocking high performance in healthcare. McKinsey&Company white paper, from McKinsey's London Office; 2009. For information, contact james_mountford@mckinsey.com.
9. Zohar D. A group-level model of safety climate: testing the effect of group climate on microaccidents in manufacturing jobs. J Appl Psychol 2000;85(4):587–96.
10. Rosen A, Singer S, Zhao S, et al. Hospital safety climate and safety outcomes: is there a relationship in the VA? Med Care Res Rev 2010;67(5):590–608.
11. Parand A, Dopson S, Renz A, et al. The role of hospital managers in quality and patients safety: a systematic review. BMJ Open 2014;4(9):e005055.

12. Millar R, Mannion R, Freeman T, et al. Hospital board oversight of quality and patient safety: a narrative review and synthesis of recent empirical research. Milbank Q 2013;91(4):738–40.
13. McFadden KL, Stock GN. Leadership, safety climate and CQI: impact on process quality and patient safety. Health Care Manage Rev 2015;40(1):24–34.
14. Grethlein SJ, Clyne B, McKean E. Leadership in health care. In: Skochelak SE, Hawkins R, Lawson L, et al, editors. Health systems science. 1st edition. Philadelphia: Elsevier; 2017. p. 92–104.
15. Burns JM. Leadership. New York: Harper & Row; 1979.
16. Bass BM, Avolio BJ. Developing transformational leadership: 1992 and beyond. J European Industrial Training 1990;14(5):21–7.
17. Quinn R. Moments of greatness: entering the fundamental state of leadership. Harv Bus Rev 2005;83(7):74–83, 191.
18. Spinelli R. The applicability of Bass's model of transformational, transactional, and laissez-faire leadership in the hospital administrative environment. Hosp Top 2006;84(2):11–9.
19. Quinn R, Rohrbaugh J. A competing values approach to organizational effectiveness. Public Productivity Review 1981;5(2):122.
20. Cameron K, Quinn R, DeGraff J, et al. Competing values leadership. Cheltenham (UK): E. Elgar Pub; 2006. p. 32.
21. National Center for Healthcare Leadership. Healthcare leadership competency model. 2006. Available at: http://www.nchl.org/documents/navlink/nchl_competency_model-full_uid892012226572.pdf. Accessed September 7, 2018.
22. Academy of Medical Royal Colleges. Medical leadership competency framework. Enhancing engagement in medical leadership. 3rd edition. London: NHS Institute for Innovation and Improvement and Academy of Medical Royal Colleges; 2011.
23. Shook J. Managing to learn. Cambridge (MA): Lean Enterprise Institute; 2008.
24. Al-Touby S. Functional results-oriented healthcare leadership: a novel leadership model. Oman Med J 2012;27(2):104–7.
25. Stefl ME. Common competencies for all healthcare managers: the Healthcare Leadership Alliance model. J Healthc Manag 2008;53(6):360–73.
26. Gillespie NA, Mann L. Transformational leadership and shared values: the building blocks of trust. J Managerial Psychology 2004;19(6):588–607.
27. Edmonson AC. Speaking up in the operating room: how team leaders promote learning in interdisciplinary action teams. J Manag Stud 2003;40(6):1419–52.
28. Kliger J. 9 essential skills of a healthcare quality improvement leader. In: Becker's Hospital review, 2013. Available at: https://www.beckershospitalreview.com/quality/9-essential-skills-of-a-healthcare-quality-improvement-leader.html. Accessed April 29, 2018.
29. Angood P, Birk S. The value of physician leadership. American College of Physician Executives white paper. Tampa (FL): American Association for Physician Leadership; 2014. Available at: https://www2.physicianleaders.org/docs/default-source/special-reports/the-value-of-physician-leadership.pdf. Accessed May 7, 2018.
30. Furtner MR, Baldegger U, Rauthmann JF. Leading yourself and leading others: linking self-leadership to transformational, transactional and laissez-faire leadership. European Journal of Work and Organizational Psychology 2013;22(4):436–49.
31. Marks MA, Mathieu JE, Zaccaro SJ. A temporally based framework and taxonomy of team processes. Acad Manag Rev 2001;26(3):356–76.

32. Ashford SJ, Sutcliffe KM, Christianson MK. Leadership, voice, and silence. In: Greenberg J, Edwards MS, editors. Voice and silence in organizations. Bingley (UK): Emerald Publishing Group; 2009. p. 175–201.

33. Hawkins JW, Fontenot HB. Mentorship: the heart and soul of health care leadership. J Healthc Leadersh 2010;2:31–4.

34. Sweeney-Platt J. Can strong leadership boost engagement? Watertown (MA): Athena Health; 2017. Available at: https://www.athenahealth.com/insight/strong-physician-leaders-key-tackling-change. Accessed May 13, 2018.

35. Johnson JK, Miller SH, Horowitz SD. Systems-based practice: improving the safety and quality of patient care by recognizing and improving the systems in which we work. In: Henriksen K, Battles JB, Keyes MA, et al, editors. Advances in patient safety: new directions and alternative approaches (Vol. 2: culture and Redesign). Rockville (MD): Agency for Healthcare Research and Quality; 2008. Available at: https://www.ncbi.nlm.nih.gov/books/NBK43731/pdf/Bookshelf_NBK43731.pdf. Accessed May 13, 2018.

36. Mann D. The missing link: lean leadership. Front Health Serv Manage 2009;26(1): 15–26.

37. A culture of change at ThedaCare. In: Institute for healthcare improvement (IHI) improvement stories. Available at: http://www.ihi.org/resources/Pages/ImprovementStories/ThedaCareFeatureStory.aspx. Accessed May 15, 2018.

38. Womack JP, Byrne AP, Fiume OJ, et al. Going lean in health care. IHI innovation series white paper. Cambridge (MA): Institute for Healthcare Improvement; 2005. Available at: http://www.ihi.org/resources/Pages/IHIWhitePapers/GoingLeaninHealthCare.aspx. Accessed November 11, 2014.

39. Meet Michigan Medicine: Quality Department. In: Michigan medicine headlines, 2017. Available at: https://www.mmheadlines.org/2017/10/meet-michigan-medicine-quality-department/. Accessed May 15, 2018.

Patient Engagement in Otolaryngology

Marisa A. Ryan, MD, MPH[a], Emily F. Boss, MD, MPH[b],*

KEYWORDS

- Patient safety • Patient engagement • Patient experience of care
- Patient-centered care • Family-centered care • Shared decision-making
- Quality improvement

KEY POINTS

- Patients and families should be integrated into health care systems to detect and prevent errors.
- Appropriate use of information technology, patient-centered communication, shared decision making, and patient experience measurement improves patient engagement.
- Patient engagement promotes safety by improving the accuracy of electronic health record data, error detection, and treatment decisions and adherence.

Patient engagement includes behaviors by patients and health professionals that promote the inclusion of patients as collaborative, active members of the care team.[1] Closely related to patient engagement, patient-centered care is characterized as "respectful of, and responsive to, individual patient preferences, needs and values, and ensuring that patient values guide all clinical decisions."[2] One approach to promote patient engagement and patient-centered care is through shared decision-making (SDM).

In addition to an emphasis on clinician–patient communication and SDM, there is increased attention to patient experience as a measure of quality health care. Patient-centered access includes availability, appropriateness, preference, and timeliness in medical care and is an important component of health care quality that is assessed on patient experience surveys.[3]

Disclosure Statement: None.
[a] Department of Otolaryngology–Head and Neck Surgery, Johns Hopkins University School of Medicine, 601 North Caroline Street, Baltimore, MD 21287, USA; [b] Departments of Otolaryngology–Head and Neck Surgery, Pediatrics, and Health Policy & Management, Johns Hopkins University School of Medicine and Bloomberg School of Public Health, 601 North Caroline Street, Baltimore, MD 21287, USA
* Corresponding author.
E-mail address: erudnic2@jhmi.edu

Otolaryngol Clin N Am 52 (2019) 23–33
https://doi.org/10.1016/j.otc.2018.08.003
0030-6665/19/© 2018 Elsevier Inc. All rights reserved.

The ideal management of medical problems requires patients to understand their own conditions and recognize that they are active participants in treatment and health maintenance. Patient engagement is enhanced through patient-centered communication, SDM, and patient experience measurement. Patient engagement can then drive improvements in patient safety (**Fig. 1**).

Since 2012, there has been an increase in research regarding patient engagement in otolaryngology.[4–10] There has also been more attention on patient-centered outcomes and patient involvement in the application of clinical research. Patients and patient representatives are now included in the American Academy of Otolaryngology-Head and Neck Surgery Foundation's (AAO-HNSF) clinical practice guidelines committees.[5]

Patient safety continues to be prioritized in otolaryngology. Shah and colleagues[11] surveyed the AAO-HNS membership in 2012 to better understand specialty-specific adverse events. Several of the identified events can be mitigated by enhanced patient engagement[11]:

- "Incomplete or incorrect history and physical," because the patient withheld information;
- "Wrong-site surgery": mark and confirm with awake patients and caregivers present;
- "Patient instructions incorrect/not followed": improve clarity and reminders of instructions;
- "Medication errors": confirm allergies and medications with patients; and
- "Physician to patient communication errors."

We discuss engagement strategies related to health information technology, patient-centered communication, SDM, and patient experience that can minimize these types of events.

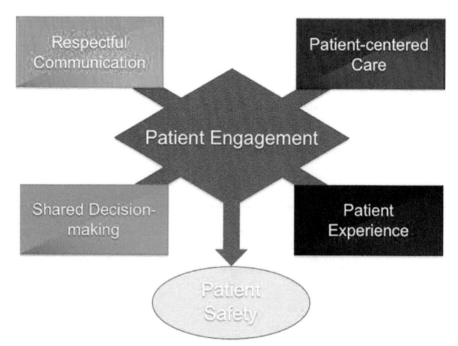

Fig. 1. Components of patient engagement that contribute to patient safety.

PATIENT ENGAGEMENT IN THE ERA OF INFORMATION TECHNOLOGY

As electronic health records (EHRs) become ubiquitous and more advanced, they have potential to work both for and against patient engagement. EHRs offer appointment reminders, preappointment/surgical communications, and postdischarge communications. These reminders have the potential to improve timely access to care, decrease missed appointments, enhance adherence to instructions, and decrease frustrations.

Patient portals and secure messaging are a relatively novel method for patient engagement that may enhance patient experience.[12,13] Lapses in medication use can be avoided with portal prescription refill requests. Patients can access portals to quickly check medications prescribed, instructions given, and next appointments. Patients can securely message the health care team when more information is needed. Although this process facilitates rapid clarifications, some patient questions require face-to-face appointments for the safest care. The clinician must recognize when that point has been reached and then bring in the patient in a timely manner. Additionally, the time and effort spent by the clinician on these communications are not consistently acknowledged through reimbursement and may place an extra burden on the clinician.[14] Moreover, patients from vulnerable populations may not have consistent access computers or health information technology.[15] It is not yet clear how portals impact the quality and safety of patient care. Although information technology is a growing component of our health system, human factors are still the basis of health care and safety.

Involving the Patient in Using the Electronic Health Record

EHRs can limit our ability to be present with the patient, but can be used effectively to enhance engagement and safety. Members of the AAO-HNS reported proportionally more errors related to EHRs in 2014 compared with 2004.[11] Some practices around EHR use can minimize these risks. Clinicians can start a visit by explaining the role of the computer and EHR and that they may be looking away at times to reference history and document.[16] Clinicians can sit to type with the screen turned so the patient can see the screen as well as their face.[16] Patient participation in building their chart can be encouraged by reading back data that are already present or that are being added. If patients seem annoyed by repetitive documentation in their EHR by multiple team members, then simple statements such as, "I am required to document this—I want to make sure we get it right for you so you receive safe care" can be used to allay their annoyance. Applying patient-centered EHR use and language in these interactions can improve patient engagement and experience.[10,17] Allowing patients easy access to the information contained in their medical records is an additional safety check that also enhances patient engagement.

Encourage Patient Engagement to Ensure Safe Care

Otolaryngologists can promote active patient engagement and additional resources are available to optimize engagement. The Agency for Healthcare Research and Quality patient involvement portal, the Joint Commission Speak Up program and the World Health Organization online toolbox offer patient brochures, infographics, and videos that focus on supporting effective patient engagement to optimize safety. Busy clinicians can make such resources available for patients to better understand effective engagement that is not confrontational and improves the safety of their care.

PATIENT-CENTERED COMMUNICATION SKILLS TO IMPROVE PATIENT ENGAGEMENT AND EXPERIENCE

Familiarity with the Patient

Clinicians, as humans, make mistakes when providing medical care. Moreover, clinicians are busy and may be pressured for time. An incomplete understanding of the patient may contribute to poor understanding and potentially harmful decision-making and treatment. Patient and family advisory councils, such as the Pediatric Family Advisory Council at Johns Hopkins Children's Center, solicit and share patient and family needs. There is a primary wish from these councils for clinicians to read and know the history of the patient before entering the room. Office systems can encourage and remind patients to send and bring relevant medical records for visits. Reviewing all available information and seeking missing data from patients can minimize harm. Additionally, highlighting important information in the medical record for other clinicians will also maximize patient safety.

Clarity, Jargon, and Complex Language

As clinicians, it may be difficult to speak without using complex medical terminology or "jargon."[18] If using jargon, it is helpful to add an explanation immediately following the term, "This study shows sleep apnea, which means there is pausing in breathing while sleeping." The framework of SDM begins with the clinician explaining information so that the patient and family can understand.[18] Calkins and colleagues[19] found that physicians overestimated their patients' understanding of the postdischarge treatment plan. Information is increasingly electronic through practice websites, patient portals, and social media platforms. The creation of complementary verbal, written, illustrated, and interactive instructions may enhance patient comprehension.[20] However, the most commonly encountered websites about pediatric otolaryngology conditions do not meet health literacy standards and include inconsistent information.[21–23] Low health literacy as well as weak clinician–patient communication have been linked to medication errors.[24]

Promotion of Patient Education

Many otolaryngologic interventions have complex posttreatment care. Within pediatric otolaryngology, tracheostomy has the highest proportion of morbidity and adverse events.[25] Thorough caregiver education, including active demonstration of acquired skills, is important to maintain safety for patients with tracheostomies. Gaudrea and colleagues[26] showed decreased complication rates after pediatric tracheostomy after the institution of a postoperative protocol for parent education. Colandrea and Eckardt[27] also showed decreased tracheostomy-related readmissions among adult veterans after creating a program in tracheostomy care and discharge education. Effective communication and teaching by the health care team can improve comprehension of instructions given and reduce errors.

Consideration of Biases

Whether or not admitted, most professionals bring to their work and interpersonal interactions a predetermined social bias. These biases consist of attitudes, beliefs, or stereotypes about people based on social group membership (eg, race, socioeconomic status, gender, religion, and sexuality) that may impact our judgment, behavior, or decisions.[28] These biases may diminish patient engagement and enhance the opportunity for errors in decision-making, because the clinician may tailor information based on preconceived perceptions of cultural needs or preferences.[28,29] This factor can affect the provision of appropriately timed follow-up, treatment adherence, and the overall safety of care.[29] Clinician bias in documentation can even diminish delivery of safe and patient-centered care by subsequent clinicians.[30] All clinicians should be trained in recognizing their own biases and work to moderate communication so that patients of all backgrounds are engaged.[28,29] More research is needed to understand the effects of these biases in otolaryngology, patient engagement, and patient safety.

SHARED DECISION-MAKING

The National Academy of Medicine defines SDM as a process in which clinicians and patients "collaborate to mutually agree on individualized health care plans for treatment and diagnostic testing."[31] There are often viable medical and surgical options to treat the same conditions in otolaryngology, for example, obstructive sleep apnea, otosclerosis, and early stage laryngeal carcinoma. SDM is most applicable when there is no single treatment option. In these situations, individual patient preferences in addition to the clinical evidence, risks, and benefits can factor more into the decision-making (**Fig. 2**). Increased patient participation in care improves adherence to treatment plans, including correct medication use and appropriate follow-up.[32] In recent years, there has been an increased emphasis on greater patient access to medical information and the use of SDM[6,12]; however, the degree to which these interventions occur in otolaryngology is variable.[18] SDM has been shown to improve health care-related decision-making quality surrounding elective surgeries[33] and specifically in otolaryngology.[20,34–36]

Decisional conflict and regret can occur during or after a health care-related decision and can be avoided through use of SDM.[20,33–36] Parents of children who snore are more satisfied with their medical care when SDM is part of the treatment process.[20] Decision aids such as option grids and scales can be used in the decision-making process. Maguire and colleagues[37] have published a visual decision aid for pediatric tonsillectomy and adenoidectomy to treat obstructive sleep apnea (**Fig. 3**). Several other communication strategies can be used to incorporate SDM in otolaryngology.

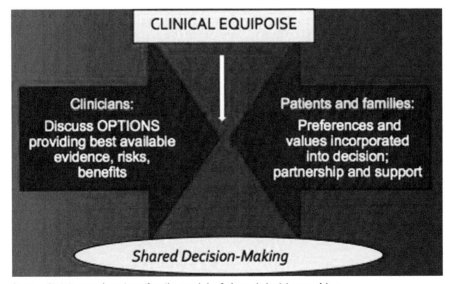

Fig. 2. Clinician and patient/family model of shared decision-making.

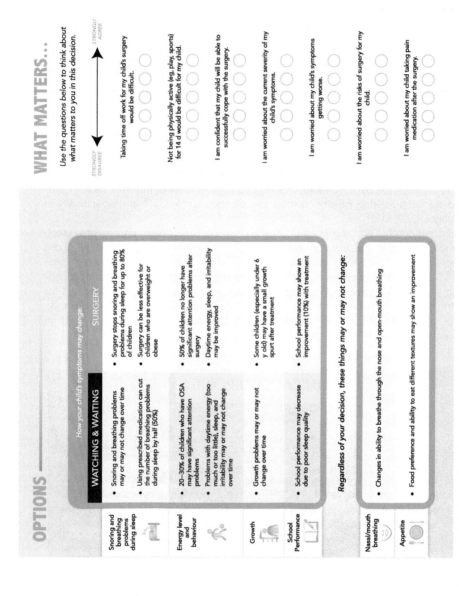

Fig. 3. Excerpt from a family decision aid for pediatric tonsillectomy and adenoidectomy to treat obstructive sleep apnea (OSA). (*From* Maguire E, Hong P, Ritchie K, et al. Decision aid prototype development for parents considering adenotonsillectomy for their children with sleep disordered breathing. J Otolaryngol Head Neck Surg 2016;45(1):57; with permission.)

Ask About Concerns and Fears

Learning patient concerns and fears provides another opportunity to engage patients as well as uncover potential areas of misunderstanding that may contribute to adverse events. Some patients and families may not feel comfortable voicing a concern or asking a question unless specifically invited. Intermittently taking pause to ask open ended questions such as, "What questions do you have for me?" and "What are you most concerned about?", can prevent patients from feeling rushed and enable them to engage as much as they are comfortable.[18,20] Especially in the inpatient setting, clinicians may not explain a treatment recommendation enough so that the patient understands and can engage in SDM.[38] In some instances, when patients raise opinions or questions, it incurs conflict with the clinicians.[38] Instead, Gulbrandsen and colleagues[39] propose that SDM should be used to foster "patient autonomy with the curating help of physicians who are attentive to patients' informational, emotional, and relational needs."

Engage Everyone

It is importance to engage patients as well as family and caretakers. Many otolaryngology patients are children or elderly with caretakers. This complexity is often compounded when more than one caregiver is involved and when assent, especially from adolescent patients, should be incorporated.[6] Allowing family and caregivers to engage when the patient cannot allows all patients to remain engaged at least by proxy.

EVALUATING PATIENT EXPERIENCE AND ENGAGEMENT TO DETECT ADVERSE EVENTS AND IMPROVE CARE DELIVERY SYSTEMS
Assessing Patient Experience

Patient experience surveys are an important measure of the health care experience and include surveys from the Consumer Assessment of Healthcare Providers and Systems (CAHPS), Press Ganey, and the National Research Corporation Health. Press Ganey and the National Research Corporation Health privately administer surveys that parallel the themes and content of the CAHPS surveys, which are overseen by Agency for Healthcare Research and Quality and Centers for Medicare and Medicaid Services. The results of these surveys are now incorporated into value-based reimbursement, clinician incentives, and public reporting initiatives. These surveys are designed to improve care delivery by identifying successes and deficiencies through patient perspectives and have become a core element of patient quality infrastructure.[7–10,40,41] These surveys can also be tapped to assess patient safety.

Active surveillance of safety events is needed for ongoing improvement in safety. Most hospital incidence reporting systems are a valuable source of safety data but are not readily open for direct patient concerns. Some of the CAHPS questions relating to safety include[41]:

- "Did anyone in this surgeon's office warn you about any signs or symptoms that would need immediate medical attention during your recovery period?"
- "Did anyone in this surgeon's office give you easy to understand instructions about what to do during your recovery period?"
- "Did providers or other hospital staff tell you how to report if you had any concerns about mistakes in your child's health care?"
- "Is there anything else you would like to say about the care your child received during this hospital stay?"

These surveys have not been used traditionally to detect errors or ongoing safety concerns, but the data collected from patient surveys can be used in this way. Weingart and colleagues[42] found an 8% incidence of self-reported adverse events and a 4% incidence of near misses in inpatient adults in the United States. None of these events were identified in the hospital incident reporting system, although 55% of the adverse events were documented in the medical record.[42] This finding suggests that adding patient-reported adverse events or near misses could increase the proportion of safety events identified and addressed. Patients can also be directly surveyed after a safety event. Millman and colleagues[43] describe an illustrative case of eliciting the patient perspective after a fall while hospitalized. If a safety event occurs, then understanding the patient's perspective can help to both support them afterward and prevent similar events in the future.

Assessing Patient Engagement

Although patient experience and engagement are interlinked, they are not the same. Patient experience surveys may reveal quality of care opportunities, but do not directly measure patient engagement. There are other validated measures for patient engagement, including the:

- Patient Activation Measure,
- Patient-Reported Outcomes Measurement Information System, and
- Patient Health Engagement Scale.

These measures have been used to assess the effect of patient engagement on quality of health care in other specialties[44,45] and can be used to improve patient engagement. Additionally, validated measures exist to assess SDM in patient interactions and these measures have been applied to otolaryngology.[46] There is also a validated measure to assess family knowledge of adenotonsillectomy and obstructive sleep apnea.[47] Incorporating these types of measures into clinical care and research could be a next step in improving patient engagement in otolaryngology.

SUMMARY

There is a shared role between clinicians and patients to improve patient engagement. There are many opportunities for clinicians and patients to work as partners toward better otolaryngology care through research, information technology, communication, and education. We should make active efforts to promote and support patient engagement while also avoiding behaviors that may inadvertently minimize patient engagement. Health care systems must be designed in a patient-centered way that also allows for the detection and prevention of errors. As the importance of patient centeredness, the patient experience, and SDM increases, otolaryngologists can also work to ensure that patient engagement concurrently improves. As patient engagement increases, this process will enable otolaryngologists and patients to improve patient safety together.

REFERENCES

1. Guide to patient and family engagement. Content last reviewed October 2014. Agency for healthcare research and quality R, MD. Available at: http://www.ahrq.gov/research/findings/final-reports/ptfamilyscan/index.html. Accessed June 30, 2018.
2. Institute of Medicine Committee on Quality of Health Care in A. Crossing the quality chasm: a new health system for the 21st century. Washington, DC: National Academies Press; 2001.

3. Berry LL, Seiders K, Wilder SS. Innovations in access to care: a patient-centered approach. Ann Intern Med 2003;139(7):568–74.
4. Pynnonen MA, Hawley ST. A patient-centered approach to clinical practice guidelines in otolaryngology. Otolaryngol Head Neck Surg 2014;150(6):910–3.
5. Roman BR, Feingold J. Patient-centered guideline development: best practices can improve the quality and impact of guidelines. Otolaryngol Head Neck Surg 2014;151(4):530–2.
6. Ikeda AK, Hong P, Ishman SL, et al. Evidence-based medicine in otolaryngology part 7: introduction to shared decision making. Otolaryngol Head Neck Surg 2018;158(4):586–93.
7. Boss EF, Thompson RE. Patient experience in outpatient pediatric otolaryngology. Laryngoscope 2012;122(10):2304–10.
8. Boss EF, Thompson RE. Patient satisfaction in otolaryngology: can academic institutions compete? Laryngoscope 2012;122(5):1000–9.
9. Boss EF, Thompson RE. Patient experience in the pediatric otolaryngology clinic: does the teaching setting influence parent satisfaction? Int J Pediatr Otorhinolaryngol 2013;77(1):59–64.
10. Espinel AG, Shah RK, Beach MC, et al. What parents say about their child's surgeon: parent-reported experiences with pediatric surgical physicians. JAMA Otolaryngol Head Neck Surg 2014;140(5):397–402.
11. Shah RK, Boss EF, Brereton J, et al. Errors in otolaryngology revisited. Otolaryngol Head Neck Surg 2014;150(5):779–84.
12. Shenson JA, Cronin RM, Davis SE, et al. Rapid growth in surgeons' use of secure messaging in a patient portal. Surg Endosc 2016;30(4):1432–40.
13. Liederman EM, Lee JC, Baquero VH, et al. Patient-physician web messaging. The impact on message volume and satisfaction. J Gen Intern Med 2005;20(1):52–7.
14. Tufano JT, Ralston JD, Martin DP. Providers' experience with an organizational redesign initiative to promote patient-centered access: a qualitative study. J Gen Intern Med 2008;23(11):1778–83.
15. Sarkar U, Karter AJ, Liu JY, et al. The literacy divide: health literacy and the use of an internet-based patient portal in an integrated health system-results from the diabetes study of northern California (DISTANCE). J Health Commun 2010; 15(Suppl 2):183–96.
16. Frankel R, Altschuler A, George S, et al. Effects of exam-room computing on clinician-patient communication: a longitudinal qualitative study. J Gen Intern Med 2005;20(8):677–82.
17. Hsu J, Huang J, Fung V, et al. Health information technology and physician-patient interactions: impact of computers on communication during outpatient primary care visits. J Am Med Inform Assoc 2005;12(4):474–80.
18. Callon W, Beach MC, Links AR, et al. An expanded framework to define and measure shared decision-making in dialogue: a 'top-down' and 'bottom-up' approach. Patient Educ Couns 2018;101(8):1368–77.
19. Calkins DR, Davis RB, Reiley P, et al. Patient-physician communication at hospital discharge and patients' understanding of the postdischarge treatment plan. Arch Intern Med 1997;157(9):1026–30.
20. Boss EF, Links AR, Saxton R, et al. Parent experience of care and decision making for children who snore. JAMA Otolaryngol Head Neck Surg 2017;143(3):218–25.
21. Harris VC, Links AR, Hong P, et al. Consulting Dr. Google: quality of online resources about tympanostomy tube placement. Laryngoscope 2018;128(2):496–501.
22. Wong K, Levi JR. Readability of pediatric otolaryngology information by children's hospitals and academic institutions. Laryngoscope 2017;127(4):E138–44.

23. Wozney L, Chorney J, Huguet A, et al. Online tonsillectomy resources: are parents getting consistent and readable recommendations? Otolaryngol Head Neck Surg 2017;156(5):844–52.
24. Lemer C, Bates DW, Yoon C, et al. The role of advice in medication administration errors in the pediatric ambulatory setting. J Patient Saf 2009;5(3):168–75.
25. Shah RK, Stey AM, Jatana KR, et al. Identification of opportunities for quality improvement and outcome measurement in pediatric otolaryngology. JAMA Otolaryngol Head Neck Surg 2014;140(11):1019–26.
26. Gaudreau PA, Greenlick H, Dong T, et al. Preventing complications of pediatric tracheostomy through standardized wound care and parent education. JAMA Otolaryngol Head Neck Surg 2016;142(10):966–71.
27. Colandrea M, Eckardt P. Improving tracheostomy care delivery: instituting clinical care pathways and nursing education to improve patient outcomes. ORL Head Neck Nurs 2016;34(1):7–16.
28. Balakrishnan KBE, Chang CW. Cognitive and implicit bias as barriers to optimal patient management. From the AAO-HNSF PSQI Committee. ENT Bulletin 2018; 37(4):13–5.
29. Boss EF, Links AR, Saxton R, et al. Physician perspectives on decision making for treatment of pediatric sleep-disordered breathing. Clin Pediatr (Phila) 2017; 56(11):993–1000.
30. P Goddu A, O'Conor KJ, Lanzkron S, et al. Do words matter? Stigmatizing language and the transmission of bias in the medical record. J Gen Intern Med 2018;33(5):685–91.
31. Institute of Medicine. Engaging patients, families, and communities. In: Best care at lower cost: the path to continuously learning health care in America. Washington, DC: National Academies Press; 2012. p. 189–226.
32. Martin LR, Williams SL, Haskard KB, et al. The challenge of patient adherence. Ther Clin Risk Manag 2005;1(3):189–99.
33. Boss EF, Mehta N, Nagarajan N, et al. Shared decision making and choice for elective surgical care: a systematic review. Otolaryngol Head Neck Surg 2016; 154(3):405–20.
34. Chorney J, Haworth R, Graham ME, et al. Understanding shared decision making in pediatric otolaryngology. Otolaryngol Head Neck Surg 2015;152(5):941–7.
35. Hong P, Gorodzinsky AY, Taylor BA, et al. Parental decision making in pediatric otoplasty: the role of shared decision making in parental decisional conflict and decisional regret. Laryngoscope 2016;126(Suppl 5):S5–13.
36. Hong P, Maguire E, Purcell M, et al. Decision-making quality in parents considering adenotonsillectomy or tympanostomy tube insertion for their children. JAMA Otolaryngol Head Neck Surg 2017;143(3):260–6.
37. Maguire E, Hong P, Ritchie K, et al. Decision aid prototype development for parents considering adenotonsillectomy for their children with sleep disordered breathing. J Otolaryngol Head Neck Surg 2016;45(1):57.
38. Berger ZD, Boss EF, Beach MC. Communication behaviors and patient autonomy in hospital care: a qualitative study. Patient Educ Couns 2017;100(8):1473–81.
39. Gulbrandsen P, Clayman ML, Beach MC, et al. Shared decision-making as an existential journey: aiming for restored autonomous capacity. Patient Educ Couns 2016;99(9):1505–10.
40. Nieman CL, Benke JR, Ishman SL, et al. Whose experience is measured? A pilot study of patient satisfaction demographics in pediatric otolaryngology. Laryngoscope 2014;124(1):290–4.

41. Consumer Assessment of Healthcare Providers and Systems (CAHPS). CAHPS information. AHRQ website. Available at: https://www.ahrq.gov/cahps/index.html. Accessed June 30, 2018.
42. Weingart SN, Pagovich O, Sands DZ, et al. What can hospitalized patients tell us about adverse events? Learning from patient-reported incidents. J Gen Intern Med 2005;20(9):830–6.
43. Millman EA, Pronovost PJ, Makary MA, et al. Patient-assisted incident reporting: including the patient in patient safety. J Patient Saf 2011;7(2):106–8.
44. Graffigna G, Barello S, Bonanomi A. The role of Patient Health Engagement Model (PHE-model) in affecting patient activation and medication adherence: a structural equation model. PLoS One 2017;12(6):e0179865.
45. Bhise V, Meyer AND, Menon S, et al. Patient perspectives on how physicians communicate diagnostic uncertainty: an experimental vignette study. Int J Qual Health Care 2018;30(1):2–8.
46. Hong P, Maguire E, Gorodzinsky AY, et al. Shared decision-making in pediatric otolaryngology: parent, physician and observational perspectives. Int J Pediatr Otorhinolaryngol 2016;87:39–43.
47. Links AR, Tunkel DE, Boss EF. Stakeholder-engaged measure development for pediatric obstructive sleep-disordered breathing: the obstructive sleep-disordered breathing and adenotonsillectomy knowledge scale for parents. JAMA Otolaryngol Head Neck Surg 2017;143(1):46–54.

The Impact of Cognitive and Implicit Bias on Patient Safety and Quality

Karthik Balakrishnan, MD, MPH[a],*, Ellis M. Arjmand, MD, MMM, PhD[b]

KEYWORDS

- Heuristic • Cognitive bias • Implicit bias • System 1 • System 2 • Metacognition

KEY POINTS

- The human mind uses shortcuts to process and respond to information.
- These shortcuts bias how one responds to data when applied inappropriately.
- Biases come in 2 main groups: cognitive and implicit.
- Both cognitive and implicit biases are innate to the human mind and cannot be eliminated; clinicians are as vulnerable as any other individuals.
- The best approach to deal with this issue appears to be recognition, metacognition, and appropriate training.

INTRODUCTION

The past 2 decades have brought increased attention to the need for improvements in quality and safety in health care. Some readers will recall an era, not long ago, in which positions such as Chief Quality Officer and Senior VP for Quality and Safety did not exist. The Institute for Healthcare Improvement (established in 1991), the National Patient Safety Foundation (established in 1997), and the landmark report "To Err is Human" from the Institute of Medicine (1999) dramatically changed the perspective of the medical community and the American public. However, improvements in quality and progress in reducing harm have not proceeded at the desired rate. For example, medical error was recently reported to be the third leading cause of death in the United States.[1]

The reality is that clinicians are *human*, with all of the attendant weaknesses and vulnerabilities that term implies. Factors, such as fatigue, burnout, high-pressure or

Disclosure: Neither author has any conflicts of interest to disclose.
[a] Department of Otolaryngology and Mayo Clinic Children's Center, Mayo Clinic College of Medicine & Science, 200 First Street Southwest, Rochester, MN 55905, USA; [b] Bobby Alford Department of Otolaryngology–Head and Neck Surgery, Texas Children's Hospital, Baylor College of Medicine, 1 Baylor Plaza, Houston, TX 77030, USA
* Corresponding author.
E-mail address: balakrishnan.karthik@mayo.edu

Otolaryngol Clin N Am 52 (2019) 35–46
https://doi.org/10.1016/j.otc.2018.08.016
0030-6665/19/© 2018 Elsevier Inc. All rights reserved.

high-risk clinical situations, and increased time and productivity pressures, all reduce the ability to provide optimal and just care to every patient. The result is inconsistent decision making that directly affects the quality of the medical care they provide. This article discusses ways in which the human mind fails to achieve perfectly rational reasoning and therefore undermines the efforts to provide the highest-quality and fairest care possible.

DIAGNOSTIC AND DECISION ERROR AS AN OBSTACLE TO HIGH-QUALITY CARE

One explanation that has been offered for the lack of accelerated improvement in quality, safety, and outcomes in health care is the lack of focus on medical decision making, particularly diagnostic error, as a cause of harm.[2,3] Although precise measures of diagnostic error are not available, some investigators have identified multiple methods for improving the identification and categorization of diagnostic errors.[2] Estimates are that the diagnostic failure rate is 10% to 15% overall, and higher in specialties such as emergency medicine in which patients are diagnostically undifferentiated. When diagnostic error occurs, cognitive factors have been implicated in a large majority of cases.[4,5]

Despite the importance of diagnostic error to patient safety, the initial focus of patient safety initiatives has been on tangible and easily addressable problems, such as procedural and medication errors,[6] and on system- and process-level problems.[7] However, individual human minds, and therefore the potential for decision errors, are still present at the interface between each step in a care process and the implementation of that step for a given patient. These diagnostic and decision errors, which are more difficult to identify, categorize, and address, form the "higher hanging fruit" of the patient safety movement. It is worth noting that errors are frequently associated with common diagnoses, for which medical knowledge is typically extensive; in such cases, judgment errors rather than knowledge deficiency is the primary issue.

COGNITIVE PROCESSES AND HEURISTICS

Concurrent with the increased attention to quality and safety in health care, in recent decades there has also been a transformation in the understanding of the psychology of decision making. The pioneering research of Amos Tversky and Daniel Kahneman,[8] which led to a Nobel Prize in Economics for Kahneman in 2002, identified various forms of systematic bias in decision making. There is now an extensive scientific literature on the various cognitive biases, also termed heuristics, and a second Nobel Prize in Economics in a closely related area was awarded to Richard Thaler in 2017. Despite these advances in the understanding of decision making in other fields, however, the literature on how heuristics affect medical decision making is relatively sparse; there has been little effort to relate systematic bias in decision making to errors that result in adverse outcomes for patients.

The essential model proposed by Kahneman, which was popularized in his 2001 book *Thinking, Fast and Slow*, involves 2 modes of cognitive processing, system 1 and system 2. System 1 is fast, efficient, and intuitive and relies heavily on heuristics, or cognitive "shortcuts." System 2 is slower, deliberative, and under conscious control. One system is not "better" than the other; rather, they serve different purposes. A simple thought experiment involving commonly occurring situations illustrates this point.

One can imagine the contrast between driving one's own car in good weather conditions on familiar roads, and the experience of driving a rental car in dangerous weather conditions in an unfamiliar city. In the first instance, an experienced driver may arrive at the destination with little memory of the journey, having relied extensively on intuitive, reflexive, system 1 decision making while driving. In the second instance, safe driving involves a more complex cognitive task: more deliberative decision making is needed; the driver must pay greater attention, and system 2 processes will be engaged. Little imagination is required to contemplate analogous scenarios in clinical medicine, some in which intuitive and efficient decision making is appropriate, and others in which a more methodical approach is preferable.

One can also imagine that an inexperienced driver would need to engage system 2 even in good weather conditions and on familiar roads. However, with increased experience, activities that once required considerable cognitive processing (system 2) can be shifted to a more reflexive and intuitive cognitive mode, which relies heavily on pattern recognition (system 1).[9] This insight is a critical insight: system 2 thinking is not "better," nor is a reliance on system 1 thinking "wrong" or dangerous, but an inappropriate reliance on heuristics and intuitive thinking in an unfamiliar or complex situation can lead to error and harm. This relationship between heuristics and error is based on the essential point that heuristics would produce predictable, systematic biases (deviations from perfectly rational thinking) when misapplied.[3]

PARTICULAR COGNITIVE CHALLENGES IN MEDICAL DECISION MAKING

Health care in particular is vulnerable to the negative effects of poor probability estimation skills. By necessity, those in health care work under constant conditions of uncertainty. The information used to make diagnoses and treatment decisions is invariably incomplete. What information one does have is of unclear accuracy, given that reliance is heavily on histories taken from patients' own unreliable recollections. Many decisions are made each day, and these decisions often carry the weight of potentially significant consequences. Furthermore, surgeons in particular may have to make many decisions under stressful or urgent circumstances. All of these factors favor an approach to "reduce the complex tasks of assessing probabilities and predicting values to simpler judgmental operations,"[8] namely heuristics.

This situation is made more complex by the various dynamics at play during clinical interactions. These dynamics can perhaps be simply classified into 3 main groups. First, there are the cognitive processes and biases through which the clinician perceives and interprets clinical data. Second, there are the implicit and social biases affecting the clinician's perception of the patient as a person, which in turn can color the clinician's interpretation. Finally, there are the patient's biases toward the clinician, which may affect the information they provide and their willingness to accept treatment recommendations. Each of these dynamics can affect the quality of the clinical interaction and the care it produces. This article will address the first 2 in particular.

COGNITIVE BIASES IN CLINICAL MEDICINE

There is a natural tendency to default to system 1 thinking in general, because it is rapid, efficient, and less taxing. This tendency is even stronger when an individual is stressed, fatigued, or under time pressure. In such circumstances, people are disinclined to accept additional uncertainty. These conditions of stress, fatigue, and time pressure are common in clinical medicine, and unfortunately, they are conditions in which deliberative decision making would appear to be even more important in order to avoid error. A study of extraneous factors in judicial decision making illustrates this effect.

Danziger and colleagues[10] reviewed more than 1000 cases in which 8 different judges evaluated petitions to grant parole. After controlling for factors such as criminal record, length of incarceration, and prisoner ethnicity, the investigators found that the likelihood of granting parole varied systematically with the time at which the case was heard. Parole was more likely to be granted (approximately 65% favorable decisions) at the start of the day, immediately after the midmorning break, and immediately after the lunch break. However, as each session progressed, the likelihood of being granted parole declined to approximately 10% before the next break was taken. The investigators found that there is a tendency to rule in favor of the status quo when making repeated rulings, and they conclude that extraneous variables ("legally irrelevant situational determinants") can influence judicial decisions. Although the findings of this study focus on legal decisions, the investigators speculate that experts involved in other important sequential decisions, such as medical decision makers, may be affected by similar decision strategies. They conclude that "the caricature that justice is what the judge ate for breakfast might be an appropriate caricature for human decision making in general." The reader can imagine a similar process affecting clinicians who are making decisions under conditions of fatigue, stress, hunger, or distraction. However, there has been little investigation of such tendencies in clinical medicine.

This section explores the application of common heuristics to decision making in medicine, with an emphasis on understanding how cognitive biases can lead to error in clinical settings. Several articles by Croskerry[3,6,11,12] have related advances in cognitive psychology to the process of decision making in medicine. Croskerry and colleagues[12] have proposed the "Dual Process Theory" model of decision making, which closely follows the system 1 and system 2 model proposed by Kahneman. This model has 8 major components, as follows:

1. Type 1 processing is fast, autonomous, largely unconscious, and uses heuristics heavily
2. Type 2 processing is slower, deliberative, and rule based and is under conscious control
3. Predictable deviations from rational decision making (*systematic biases*) that lead to error occur more frequently with type 1 processes
4. Repetitive utilization of type 2 may allow for eventual processing in type 1 for a given situation (this represents skill acquisition)
5. Biases affecting decision making in type 1 processing can be "overridden" by explicit effort to use type 2 processing. This is the basis of debiasing using metacognition
6. Excessive reliance on type 1 processing can override type 2 processing, leading to unexamined decisions
7. Decision makers can move rapidly between type 1 and type 2 processes
8. There is a tendency to default to type 1 processing when possible ("cognitive miser" effect)

When using system 1, or when engaged in type 1 processing, one relies on cognitive biases or heuristics. Some of these were described by Kahneman and Tversky in their early publications, and the list of known biases has been expanded by subsequent research. Elstein[13] summarized selected errors in clinical reasoning and considered biases in diagnostic reasoning and biases in treatment separately, as follows:

Biases in Diagnostics Reasoning

1. Judgment affected by ease of recall: the tendency to overestimate the frequency of easily recalled events and underestimate the frequency of ordinary or difficult to recall events (also referred to as the *availability heuristic*)

2. Judging by similarity: the tendency to estimate probability based on similarity to diagnostic category or prototype, without considering base rates (also referred to as the *representativeness heuristic*)
3. Conservatism: the failure to revise diagnostic possibilities sufficiently when presented with new information, resulting in a tendency to collect more data than are needed (also referred to as *anchoring and adjustment*)
4. Acquiring redundant evidence: the tendency to seek information that confirms a hypothesis rather than information that *tests* a competing hypothesis (also referred to as *confirmation bias*)
5. Anchoring and adjustment: the tendency for the final diagnosis to be closer to the initial diagnosis that would be implied by rational assessment of the clinical evidence
6. Order effects: the tendency for final opinions to be affected by the order in which information is received, giving more weight to information presented early in the case (*primacy*) or late in a case (*recency*)

Biases in Treatment

1. Omission bias: the tendency of experienced physicians to recommend treatment less frequently than their own models would suggest. This bias against action (bias in favor of omission) appears to be related to a feeling that harm as a result of treatment is worse than harm that results from no treatment
2. Outcome bias: the tendency to assess the quality of a decision based on outcomes rather than on the logic of the decision process

Elstein called for increased awareness of these processes by physicians and medical educators as an important strategy for minimizing effects that result from their misapplication, stating, "as with visual illusions, awareness does not prevent us from being susceptible to their effects, but we can know that we are being fooled. Similarly, awareness of the limitations of human judgment can lead to more thoughtful deliberations, which in turn will enhance the quality of decision making."

Some investigators have expressed reservations about the stigma associated with using the word "bias" to describe what are essentially normal cognitive processes. *Cognitive dispositions to respond*, or *CDRs*, has been proposed as an alternative term describing the normal tendency to respond to situations in predictable ways.[11] Some common CDRs that can lead to diagnostic errors are as follows:

1. Anchoring: the tendency to establish a diagnosis too early in the diagnostic process, and failing to adjust the initial impression in consideration of additional information
2. Availability: the tendency to assess something as more likely if it comes easily to mind, such as when a condition has been seen recently
3. Base-rate neglect: the tendency to ignore the true prevalence of a disease or condition when evaluating the probability of its presence in an individual patient
4. Confirmation bias: the tendency to accept confirmatory evidence more readily than disconfirming evidence
5. Frame blindness: the tendency to be overly influenced by the way in which a question is framed; may result in providing the "right answer to the wrong question"
6. Gambler's fallacy: the belief that the probability of a patient having a diagnosis is influenced by independent preceding events
7. Hindsight bias: the influence of knowing the outcome on the perception of past events

8. Order effects: the tendency to remember initial events (primacy) or the last events (recency)
9. Outcome bias: the tendency to opt for what one hopes will happen rather than what is most likely to happen
10. Overconfidence bias: the tendency to believe that one knows more than they do. This effect is augmented by anchoring and by availability
11. Premature closure: the tendency to arrive at a diagnosis before it has been verified
12. Sunk costs: the tendency to remain attached to a diagnosis that one is invested in, and a reluctance to consider alternative. May be influenced by confirmation bias
13. Vertical line failure: routine tasks and predictable styles that emphasize economy and utility, and the failure to consider "what else could this be?"

A commonly used method for describing the impact of cognitive biases, heuristics, or CDRs on medical decision making is to analyze a clinical case involving a missed diagnosis using these concepts. The published examples are generally from the fields of emergency medicine and internal medicine.[14,15] Clinical examples in otolaryngology to illustrate these concepts are presented as follows.

Case 1

A 2-year-old child presented to the Emergency Department of a community hospital after a witnessed choking episode with a Lego in his mouth. The parents reported that the child had "swallowed a Lego." At the time of evaluation, the child was breathing comfortably and in stable condition. The child was transferred to the local children's hospital for further evaluation with the reported diagnosis of esophageal foreign body.

At the children's hospital, the child was breathing comfortably and swallowing without difficulty. He had mild midsternal discomfort but was otherwise asymptomatic. Chest radiographs were normal. The surgical service on call for esophageal foreign bodies was contacted, and discharge to home with primary care follow-up was recommended.

Two weeks later, the child returned with cough, fever, and noisy breathing. Evaluation revealed a tracheal foreign body. Bronchoscopy was performed, and the foreign body was removed.

Case 1 commentary This case reveals deficiencies in communication, which is a nearly universal finding in cases with adverse outcome. In addition, reviewing this case using the concepts of cognitive bias and heuristics reveals several other problems. The description by the parents that the child had "swallowed a Lego" became a point of *anchoring* for the physicians and staff. This diagnosis became "sticky," which has been described as *diagnostic momentum*: a provisional diagnosis is repeated until it becomes certain, and other possibilities are excluded. Consulting a service that manages a specific problem (esophageal foreign bodies) is an example of *triage cueing*. The question became "Is this object still in the esophagus?" rather than "Where is the foreign body that this child placed in his mouth?," which is a *framing effect*. The result was *premature closure* of the decision-making process.

This case also illustrates that diagnostic error occurs with common clinical diagnoses. In these cases, error and harm result from judgment rather than a deficiency in medical knowledge.

Case 2

A medically complex 17-year-old patient with a long-term tracheostomy and home ventilator management presented to the primary care physician's office with dyspnea and increased work of breathing. The patient had been discharged from the hospital 2 weeks earlier after a prolonged hospital stay for abdominal surgery followed by pneumonia. She was referred from the primary care provider (PCP) office to Otolaryngology with suspected mucous plugging of the airway and taken urgently to the operating room where this finding was confirmed and treated. Postoperatively, she was in stable condition in the recovery room. She was discharged to home later that day with continuation of home nursing support.

On the first morning after surgery, the patient again developed severe respiratory distress with poor air exchange through the tracheostomy tube. Attempts to clear the airway by suctioning were unsuccessful. The tracheostomy tube was changed without difficulty, but the patient still could not be ventilated. The patient was emergently transported to the hospital, where airway obstruction by extensive mucous plugging was identified. A severe hypoxic brain injury was diagnosed, and care was withdrawn.

Case 2 commentary A review of the second case reveals some similarities to the first. Problems with communication were revealed: information transfer from the PCP to the otolaryngology service was limited, and it is unclear whether the Otolaryngology physicians were aware or informed of the length, complexity, or details of the recent hospitalization. The *framing effect* is also apparent in this case, in that the focus was on clearing the airway, and the question of why this patient with no prior history of mucous plugging had now developed this problem was not addressed. *Search satisfying* is the tendency to stop looking once something has been found, which can lead to second diagnoses and comorbidities being missed. In this case, the patient had recently been hospitalized and the family strongly desired to go home, a wish that may have influenced the medical decision making. The influence of affective sources of error on decision making has been described as *visceral bias*.

> *It seems clear that how physicians think and not what physicians know is primarily responsible for diagnostic failure*
>
> —*Croskerry 2012*[6]

Despite major advances in understanding the psychology of decision making, and highly influential research demonstrating systematic forms or bias in decision making, decision theorists in medicine have largely adhered to a normative model that is somewhat removed from practical situations. The impact of cognitive biases, heuristics, or CDR in medical decision making has been largely unexplored.

There is an association between cognitive bias and diagnostic error. As described above, and in other studies, diagnostic error often occurs in common clinical situations whereby knowledge deficiencies do not appear to be the primary issue. Although the incidence of diagnostic error is difficult to establish, there is an association between these errors and patient harm. The lack of focus on cognition in medical decision making may partly explain why more rapid progress has not been made in reducing medical error.

Education and training on the psychology of decision making, metacognition (mindfulness), and the use of common terminology to describe cognitive processes are essential to understanding and reducing harm, and improving patient safety.

IMPLICIT BIAS IN CLINICAL MEDICINE

As described in the previous section, the mind's natural tendency is to rely on system 1 thinking, interpreting data through heuristics and by making rapid connections to previously available data and experiences. Beyond the CDR that affect how clinicians interpret clinical data, heuristics and systematic biases exist in how we perceive other humans, including patients. We speculate that the cognitive pathways that allow such biases may have developed to provide rapid determination of "in-group" and "out-group" status for social and reproductive purposes. However, the specifics of how we perceive other individuals, and of how we understand and classify them based on their perceivable characteristics (ie, social and cultural biases), are most likely shaped by the circumstances in which we develop.[16] Physicians are not immune to these tendencies and appear to parallel the general population in these patterns.[17]

Accordingly, the current literature suggests that social biases appear to develop early in childhood.[18] These interindividual and intergroup biases may manifest as open racism, sexism, homophobia, and other forms of discrimination; such examples are termed *explicit bias*. More commonly, they appear as *implicit bias* (sometimes called *unconscious bias*), affecting interpersonal interactions in more subtle ways of which we are not consciously aware. Interestingly, young children appear to have concordance between their self-rated and implicit biases, at least for race bias, whereas older children and adults tend to express less biased explicit views, whereas their implicit biases remain unchanged.[18] These implicit attitudes may have important health and behavioral effects. For example, implicit attitudes about tobacco use may be associated with both future smoking behaviors and future quitting.[19]

Many dimensions of implicit bias exist. Common directions along which these biases manifest are listed in later discussion. The reader will notice that all of these may be perceptible (or evaluable, although perhaps not accurately) during the first moments of any interpersonal interaction (**Box 1**).

As with the cognitive biases discussed earlier, these patterns of bias are systematic, and they may have profound effects on the quality of care one provides. Indeed, Zestcott and colleagues[17] argue that implicit biases are a major contributor to health disparities. Examples of these biases in health care abound. A recent systematic review identified 42 studies assessing implicit bias in health care providers, mostly focusing on race.[20] The investigators concluded that clinicians had a similar degree of implicit bias as the general population. Meanwhile, experimental studies have demonstrated repeatedly that these biases measurably affect clinical assessments and treatment decision making.[21] This effect appears to be particularly relevant in challenging or ambiguous situations[22] or under heavier cognitive loads,[23] as is the case with the cognitive biases discussed earlier. In turn, these biases appear to affect how patients perceive clinical encounters, driving patient satisfaction and confidence in their care.[24]

Box 1
Common dimensions of implicit bias

1. Race or ethnicity
2. Gender
3. Age
4. Sexual orientation
5. Weight
6. Education
7. Socioeconomic status
8. Tobacco and alcohol use status

If these patient effects occur during childhood, they may even have lifelong effects on health outcomes.[25]

The literature on implicit bias effects in otolaryngology is nonexistent. However, one study of 215 surgeons included 15 otolaryngologists and demonstrated that although surgeons had measurable biases, these were not associated with treatment decisions in multivariate analysis.[26] Other investigators, however, have reviewed the literature and found evidence for differential surgical treatment decisions, care quality, and outcomes when patients are compared by race.[27] The critical lesson is that health care providers and surgeons are as vulnerable to the effects of implicit bias as any other group, and that implicit bias directly prevents them from achieving the ideal of justice (fairness) in health care. The reader should keep in mind that although most examples here are race based due to the focus on race in the literature, implicit biases can work along any of the axes listed above, and many more beyond.

Every provider hopes to deliver high-quality care to every patient, but each provider's unique background and experiences may make this goal more or less elusive with each patient. These variations are specific to every provider-patient interaction. For example, perspectives can be inappropriately based on the surgeon's prior encounters with a few patients or families from a particular geographic area or cultural/ethnic group. In other words, the surgeon develops a *heuristic* connecting this ethnic group with those characteristics. One can imagine, for example, a situation in which a surgeon's unfavorable views of a particular ethnic group leads to their blaming a complication on a caregiver of different ethnicity because "those people never follow directions." A more appropriate response might be to consider what language and cultural factors might have prevented adherence to the surgeon's instructions. Perhaps an interpreter did not accurately convey the necessary information due to linguistic differences between English and the patient's preferred language; perhaps cultural factors outweighed the parent's willingness to follow medical recommendations, or perhaps the caregiver has had negative interactions with surgeons in the past and has experienced a loss of trust in them. As with cognitive biases, the provider likely has adequate clinical knowledge but might allow implicit biases to dominate decision making while under a heavy cognitive load (for example, during a busy clinic with multiple competing cognitive demands).

ADDRESSING COGNITIVE AND IMPLICIT BIAS IN HEALTH CARE

Given that cognitive and implicit biases result from misapplied or inappropriate heuristics, strategies to reduce their effects are also shared. The first and most important step is awareness that such biases exist, and recognition that every human mind uses these cognitive shortcuts. This step required "metacognition," or conscious awareness of one's own thought processes and biases. The results of this step alone appear to be mixed. In a review of the literature, Zestcott and colleagues[17] suggest that simple awareness may lead clinicians to deal with their implicit bias but that awareness strategies may also lead to defensiveness and denial. In contrast, an experimental study demonstrated that awareness of implicit bias had profound effects on physician's treatment patterns, and that most participants thought that increased awareness would improve the quality of the care they provided.[28] It is evident that few surgeons make the effort to investigate these biases in themselves,[29] suggesting that there is room for improvement.

Beyond awareness alone, cognitive biases may be addressed through active "debiasing" strategies. The logic and specifics of these approaches have been described in detail by Croskerry and colleagues.[12,30] In brief, the objective is to facilitate a switch from system 1 to system 2 through "cognitive forcing"[31] to ensure a systematic and maximally rational analysis of any clinical situation. Although studies demonstrating benefits of this approach are lacking,[32] the approach has face validity and warrants further study.

Similar "debiasing" approaches have been discussed for implicit bias. On the conceptually simplest level, Hisam and colleagues[33] recommend increased use of shared decision making and cultural humility on the part of surgeons. They also mention the value of formal statements from professional governing bodies, awareness of which seems to correlate with increased recognition of implicit biases among surgeons.[29] On a higher level, it appears that pursuit of common ground is beneficial for clinician-patient relationships that are discordant in race, gender, and other dimensions.[17] Related strategies include consciously taking the other's perspective and training the mind to see patients as individuals by eliciting counterstereotypic data. These latter strategies appear to be particularly effective, and a multipronged approach may be the most beneficial in both the short and the long term.[17] However, formal studies of the effects of these interventions remain a gap in the medical and surgical literature.

Beyond provider-patient interaction, implicit biases can also significantly affect interprovider dynamics. Society as a whole has seen a rapid increase in reporting and awareness of gender bias; for example, and medicine and otolaryngology are not exempt.[34] This bias appears to contribute to differences in career trajectory and traditional measures of academic success.[35,36] Although the same strategies of seeking individualization in small specialties such as otolaryngology, exposure to "other" groups and counterstereotypic exposures to counter such biases may be more challenging to come by. The American Academy of Otolaryngology–Head and Neck Surgery, for example, reports as of March 2018 that 17% of members self-reported female gender, and 9.5% self-reported a specific minority (personal communication, Karthik Balakrishnan, MD, MPH, 2018). These data are challenging to interpret due to the drawbacks of self-reporting and because many members declined to report a gender or ethnicity (9% and 51%, respectively), but they suggest that particularly in this specialty, clinicians must be willing to invest adequate effort to achieve any meaningful improvement in the impact of implicit biases.

SUMMARY

Cognitive and implicit bias are likely the result of ancient evolutionary processes that have created a tendency for the human mind to use cognitive shortcuts, or heuristics, which was indeed probably necessary for survival. When applied inappropriately, these heuristics lead to nonrational interpretations of available data, whether clinical or related to the patient as an individual. No clinician is exempt from these processes and their attendant risks. Accordingly, the most effective approach to minimize their effects on quality of care is likely to recognize that they exist and to pursue active debiasing measures. Although these efforts demand conscious effort and energy, available data suggest that they may have important effects in improving provider-patient interactions, quality of care, and health outcomes.

REFERENCES

1. Makary MA, Daniel M. Medical error – the third leading cause of death in the US. BMJ 2016;353:i2139.
2. Graber ML. The incidence of diagnostic error in medicine. BMJ Qual Saf 2013; 22(Suppl 2):ii21–7.

3. Croskerry P. From mindless to mindful practice — cognitive bias and clinical decision making. N Engl J Med 2013;368:2445–8.
4. Graber ML, Franklin N, Gordon R. Diagnostic error in internal medicine. Arch Intern Med 2005;165:1493–9.
5. Zwaan L, de Brujine M, Wagner C, et al. Patient record review of the incidence, consequences, and causes of diagnostic adverse events. Arch Intern Med 2010; 170:1015–21.
6. Croskerry P. Perspectives on diagnostic failure and patient safety. Healthc Q 2012;15(Spec No):50–6.
7. Reason J. Human error: models and management. BMJ 2000;320:768–70.
8. Tversky A, Kahneman D. Judgment under uncertainty: heuristics and biases. Science 1974;185:1124–31.
9. Patel VL, Kaufman DR, Arocha JF. Emerging paradigms of cognition in medical decision-making. J Biomed Inform 2002;35:52–75.
10. Danziger S, Levav J, Avnaim-Pesso L. Extraneous factors in judicial decisios. Proc Natl Acad Sci U S A 2011;108:6889–92.
11. Croskerry P. The importance of cognitive errors in diagnosis and strategies to minimize them. Acad Med 2003;78:775–80.
12. Croskerry P, Singhal G, Mamede S. Cognitive debiasing 1: origins of bias and theory of debiasing. BMJ Qual Saf 2013;22(Suppl 2):ii58–64.
13. Elstein AS. Heuristics and biases: selected errors in clinical reasoning. Acad Med 1999;74:791–4.
14. Croskerry P. Our better angels and black boxes. Emerg Med J 2016;33:242–4.
15. Redelmeier DA. The cognitive psychology of missed diagnoses. Ann Intern Med 2005;142:115–20.
16. Bigler RS, Liben LS. A developmental intergroup theory of social stereotypes and prejudice. Adv Child Dev Behav 2006;34:39–89.
17. Zestcott CA, Blair IV, Stone J. Examining the presence, consequences, and reduction of implicit bias in health care: a narrative review. Group Process Intergroup Relat 2016;19:528–42.
18. Baron AS, Banaji MR. The development of implicit attitudes: evidence of race evaluations from ages 6 and 10 and adulthood. Psychol Sci 2006;17:53–8.
19. Macy JT, Chassin L, Presson CC, et al. Changing implicit attitudes toward smoking: results from a web-based approach-avoidance practice intervention. J Behav Med 2015;38:143–52.
20. FitzGerald C, Hurst S. Implicit bias in healthcare professionals: a systematic review. BMC Med Ethics 2017;18:19.
21. Plaisime MV, Malebranche DJ, Davis AL, et al. Healthcare providers' formative experiences with race and black male patients in urban hospital environments. J Racial Ethn Health Disparities 2017;4:1120–7.
22. Hirsh AT, Hollingshead NA, Ashburn-Nardo L, et al. The interaction of patient race, provider bias, and clinical ambiguity on pain management decisions. J Pain 2015;16:558–68.
23. Johnson TJ, Hickey RW, Switzer GE, et al. The impact of cognitive stressors in the emergency department on physician implicit racial bias. Acad Emerg Med 2016; 23:297–305.
24. Penner LA, Dovidio JF, Gonzalez R, et al. The effects of oncologist implicit racial bias in racially discordant oncology interactions. J Clin Oncol 2016;34:2874–80.
25. Lang KR, Dupree CY, Kon AA, et al. Calling out implicit racial bias as a harm in pediatric care. Camb Q Healthc Ethics 2016;25:540–52.

26. Haider AH, Schneider EB, Sriram N, et al. Unconscious race and social class bias among acute care surgical clinicians and clinical treatment decisions. JAMA Surg 2015;15:457–64.

27. Torain MJ, Maragh-Bass AC, Dankwa-Mullen I, et al. Surgical disparities: a comprehensive review and new conceptual framework. J Am Coll Surg 2016; 223:408–18.

28. Green AR, Carney DR, Pallin DJ, et al. Implicit bias among physicians and its prediction of thrombolysis decisions for black and white patients. J Gen Intern Med 2007;22:1231–8.

29. Britton BV, Nagarajan N, Zogg CK, et al. Awareness of racial/ethnic disparities in surgical outcomes and care: factors affecting acknowledgement and action. Am J Surg 2016;212:102–8.

30. Croskerry P, Singhal G, Mamede S. Cognitive debiasing 2: impediments to and strategies for change. BMJ Qual Saf 2013;22(Suppl 2):ii65–72.

31. Croskerry P. Cognitive forcing strategies in clinical decision making. Ann Emerg Med 2003;41:110–20.

32. Oliver G, Oliver G, Body R. BET 2: poor evidence on whether teaching cognitive debiasing, or cognitive forcing strategies, lead to a reduction in errors attributable to cognition in emergency medicine students or doctors. Emerg Med J 2017;34:553–4.

33. Hisam B, Zogg CK, Chaudhary MA, et al. From understanding to action: interventions for surgical disparities. J Surg Res 2016;200:560–78.

34. Appold K. Otolaryngology's #MeToo: gender bias and sexual harassment in medicine. Available at: http://www.enttoday.org/article/otolaryngologys-metoo-gender-bias-and-sexual-harassment-in-medicine/. Accessed April 29, 2018.

35. Eloy JA, Mady IJ, Svider PF, et al. Regional differences in gender promotion and scholarly productivity in otolaryngology. Otolaryngol Head Neck Surg 2014;150: 371–7.

36. Eloy JA, Svider PF, Kovalerchik O, et al. Gender differences in successful NIH grant funding in otolaryngology. Otolaryngol Head Neck Surg 2013;149:77–83.

Rethinking Morbidity and Mortality Conference

Brian Nussenbaum, MD, MHCM[a,*], Richard A. Chole, MD, PhD[b]

KEYWORDS

- Morbidity and mortality conference • Otolaryngology • Just culture • Patient safety
- Quality improvement

KEY POINTS

- An effective morbidity and mortality (M&M) conference can drive the evolution of a supportive, blame-free, patient safety culture that is proactive to preventing future patient harms.
- There are key elements to an effective M&M conference and some that are counterproductive.
- Leadership support with M&M conference redesign efforts is critically important.

INTRODUCTION

Going back to the Harvard Medical Practice Study reported in 1991,[1] it is known that adverse events occur in approximately 4% of hospitalizations and that nearly 60% of these events are preventable. In otolaryngology departments, these adverse events are frequently reported through a monthly morbidity and mortality (M&M) conference, which has traditionally been an important cornerstone conference for surgical departments. Yet, these conferences can be riddled with recall bias that leads to incomplete reporting, reluctance bias caused by a "blame and shame" culture, and ineffective outputs. This article will address how the M&M conference can be used as a vehicle for advancing patient safety/quality improvement (PSQI) and minimizing conference characteristics that are counterproductive toward this goal. Key elements will be discussed that reinforce a supportive patient safety culture. These include standardized indicators for case reporting, defined mechanisms for reporting, conference organization, case selection, case analysis, and focused outputs to prevent future patient

Disclosure Statement: The authors do not have any relevant financial conflicts of interest related to this work. B. Nussenbaum is an employee of the American Board of Otolaryngology. The content of this article reflects the thoughts of the authors and not any official recommendations or positions from the American Board of Otolaryngology.
[a] American Board of Otolaryngology, 5615 Kirby Drive, Suite 600, Houston, TX 77098, USA;
[b] Department of Otolaryngology, Washington University in St. Louis, School of Medicine, 660 South Euclid Avenue, Campus Box 8115, St Louis, MO 63110, USA
* Corresponding author.
E-mail address: bn@aboto.org

harms. Innovations to augment case discussions and learning during conference will also be discussed.

TRADITIONAL MORBIDITY AND MORTALITY CONFERENCES

Many surgeons can remember attending M&M conferences during surgical training, and perhaps still currently in their workplaces, where the purpose is somewhat unclear. The characteristics of the traditional M&M conference can easily lead one to believe that the purpose is for punishment and remediation of the surgeon for having a bad outcome that may or may not have been in his or her control. The focus tends to be on the specific incident and individual rather than the faulty systems within which surgeons work. This leads directly to a "blame and shame" culture rather than a learning culture and meaningful changes. Going back to 1989, Berwick described that most problems in organizations do not come from individuals but rather from the structure of faulty systems, and that pushing people to "try harder" or "do better" will generally not result in improved performance or outcomes.[2]

Another characteristic of traditional M&M conferences includes having a single source of nonstandardized inputs and lack of transparent outputs. In academic departments, this single source is frequently residents. The combination of hierarchy, lack of reporting protocols, and a "blame and shame" culture leads to several deterrents to reporting events for the M&M conference, including reluctance bias, recall bias, and fear. The lack of outputs is particularly problematic when there are cases rooted in systems problems that require correction. Also problematic is when a system problem is fixed, but no follow-up is communicated to the conference participants. Traditional M&M conferences are usually conducted in individual departments (silos) with little interaction among various disciplines.

The characteristics described of the traditional M&M conference are not supportive of a healthy PSQI culture. A healthy patient safety culture is one that fosters high levels of trust and personal accountability, facilitates early identification of unsafe conditions, strengthens systems proactively, and regularly assesses areas of the culture needing improvement.[3] In the "11 Tenets of a Safety Culture" described by The Joint Commission, the first is "apply a transparent, nonpunitive approach to reporting and learning from adverse events, close calls, and unsafe conditions."[4] For surgical departments, this is perhaps best accomplished by rethinking the design of M&M conference. This conference is a logical vehicle for affecting safety culture change, because so many expected norms of behavior are directly translated into all aspects of this conference. To make this change, however, there needs to be collective recognition and genuine motivation for change, including strong support from leadership.

REDESIGN OF THE MORBIDITY AND MORTALITY CONFERENCE
Role of Leadership

Leadership has an enduring, critically important role throughout all phases of M&M conference redesign, but particularly early during the roll-out.

Leadership needs to create a clear sense of legitimacy and visible strong support within the department and the organization. Some actions that can contribute to this include the following:

1. Conference attendance made mandatory for all clinicians.
2. The conference name is changed to better reflect the purpose. An example might be "PSQI/M&M Conference." In some states, M&M needs to remain in the name of the conference for the case discussions to remain legally protected.

3. The assigned conference moderator is a respected, clinical leader, someone who is an influencer. This can be a formal or informal leader, but ideally would be the individual in the department responsible more globally for the department PSQI program and have a formal title to reflect this key role. This individual should have the opportunity to obtain formal training in the science and practice of PSQI rather than solely on the job learning. An appropriate level of administrative support should be provided.

Leadership needs to faithfully attend and clearly communicate commitments to all members of the department about psychological safety, which is feeling safe from retaliation, humiliation, and disrespectful behavior. These goals can be achieved by endorsing the following:

1. Applying James Reason's Swiss cheese model for case analysis when looking for root causes of adverse events and errors.[5] This commonly used tool in many industries defines the protections between a hazard and a harm, the defects (holes) in each layer of protection, which holes are related to personal versus systems factors, and how the holes (active and system failures) line up to lead to an adverse event or error.
2. Applying a "Just Culture" approach to case discussions.[6] A Just Culture is one in which individuals are held accountable for their actions but not for system flaws. This establishes an appropriate balance between a punitive culture versus a blame-free culture.
3. Applying the substitution test.[7] This is done by simply asking if the same actions or outcomes would have happened if the evaluating were instead involved with the patient's care. This tool introduces a humility element to case analysis.

Design a Structure to the Process

The timeline of an adverse event or medical error is shown in **Fig. 1**. Once the event occurs, the first step is reporting. Without consistent and robust reporting, it is difficult to know where the opportunities exist for improving quality and patient safety. Changing a reporting culture is perhaps the most difficult aspect to culture change and highly dependent on the individuals feeling psychologically safe and knowing expectations. It is important for anyone in the department to be able to report an adverse event on both the inpatient and outpatient sides. Beyond who submits reports, other important details include what to report, when to report, and how to report. In terms of what to report, it is helpful for leadership to develop trigger criteria to help guide event reporting. This list would not be all inclusive but would include the events that leadership expects should always be reported. Examples could be intraoperative mortalities, unplanned readmissions within 30 days of discharge, and unplanned reoperations within 30 days of initial surgery. It is important to emphasize the need to report near misses. These are cases when the adverse event or error does not reach the patient either because of timely intervention or by chance alone. Near misses usually have a lot to learn from but are typically under-reported, because the clinician usually makes a sigh of relief and then moves on. In terms of when to report, it is best to submit once the event occurs and then provide an update upon discharge or closure to the event. This proactive approach minimizes the recall bias that occurs when retrospectively trying to remember events from the prior month. In terms of how to report, this is done either using a departmental/institutional electronic reporting system or paper forms. Regardless of the platform used, the process for submitting cases should be simple, easy, straight-forward, and standardized.

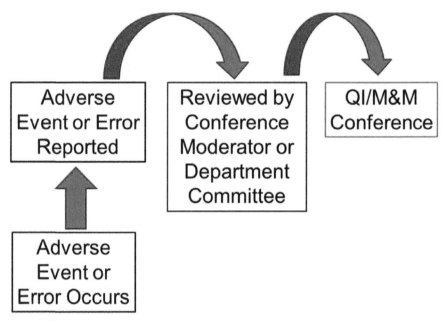

Fig. 1. Lifetime of an adverse event.

The frequent design of the M&M conference includes all reported cases being on the agenda for subsequent discussion. The problem with this approach is the limited time for conference, which is usually 1 hour in length. If there are 10 to 15 cases reported in a month, then the time availability for the conference does not allow for an in-depth, focused discussion of the few cases that truly require the most attention and have the most for everyone to learn from. Case selection and prioritization prior to the conference, performed by the conference moderator or by a department committee, helps guide which cases to focus upon during the conference. Depending on the details of the cases, it can be difficult to thoroughly discuss more than 3 to 4 cases in 1 hour.

The M&M conference structure should be standardized, with the details decided based on what works best for the local environment. The variables to consider include:

1. What is the recurring time and day each month for the conference?
2. Who are the expected attendees for the conference?
3. Which clinical sites are covered?
4. What is the conference format? One format to consider includes "New News," followed by "Closing the Loop," followed by a dashboard summary of all cases reported from all included clinical sites, followed by a detailed discussion of the prioritized cases to thoroughly discuss.
5. What is the derivation of cases? Ideally this would be from prospectively compiled case lists. It could also include hospital triggered case reviews and referrals from other departments.
6. Is there a prioritization scheme for case discussion? One protocol to consider is prioritization for discussion of mortalities related to the care delivered by the service, events categorized by the hospital as requiring a debriefing or root cause analysis,

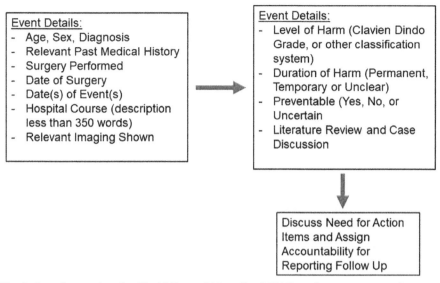

Event Details:
- Age, Sex, Diagnosis
- Relevant Past Medical History
- Surgery Performed
- Date of Surgery
- Date(s) of Event(s)
- Hospital Course (description less than 350 words)
- Relevant Imaging Shown

Event Details:
- Level of Harm (Clavien Dindo Grade, or other classification system)
- Duration of Harm (Permanent, Temporary or Unclear)
- Preventable (Yes, No, or Uncertain
- Literature Review and Case Discussion

Discuss Need for Action Items and Assign Accountability for Reporting Follow Up

Fig. 2. Sample template for Morbidity and Mortality (M&M) conference presentations.

near misses, events believed to be preventable, and events felt to have the greatest learning impact.

7. Who presents the case? In training environments, this is frequently the most senior level resident involved with the event. But sometimes because of the delicate nature of the event, it would be the attending physician.

8. Is there a template for case presentation? Use of a template decreases the chances of important information being omitted and standardizes collection of important information such as level of harm (using Clavien-Dindo grade[8] or another classification system), duration of harm (permanent, temporary, or unclear), and preventability (yes, no, or uncertain). When appropriate, use of an anonymous audience response system can further reinforce learning from a case and emphasize key concepts. An example of a presentation template is shown in **Fig. 2**.

9. Are any outputs or action items needed, and if so, who is responsible? These outputs can vary from communications with other departments to initiating systems changes to complex PSQI projects. These items go on to the Closing the Loop section for the subsequent M&M conferences until resolution/closure is reported. This provides for internal accountability and department members typically find the follow up gratifying. Keeping track of "what has changed" and giving an annual summary presentation is also a compelling communication approach to convey the effectiveness of the redesigned conference.

Particularly in an otolaryngology-head and neck surgery practice, adverse events may also involve other specialties such as anesthesia, neurosurgery, ophthalmology, thoracic surgery, and emergency medicine. In certain situations, having a joint M&M conference to discuss specific cases might be helpful if both departments plan to present the case and the culture of the departments support this approach. If there are cultural or time impediments, then alternatively it can be helpful for representation from the other service to be present during the case presentation to provide their specialty's perspective on the event.

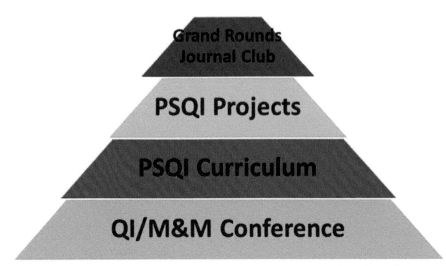

Fig. 3. Foundational effect of an effective Morbidity and Mortality (M&M) Conference.

MEASURES OF EFFECTIVENESS

There are several metrics that can be considered to measure effectiveness of the redesign of the M&M conference. An annual, anonymous survey on safety culture can be performed, with results tracked. There are several validated surveys that can be used, including the Safety Climate Scale and the AHRQ Patient Safety Culture Survey.[9,10] The number of adverse events reported yearly can be tracked. The number of PSQI projects being performed can be tracked. Lastly, the surveys can be designed to measure the effectiveness of the M&M conference. These are just a few examples of what can be used. Whatever is chosen, it is important to get baseline measurements before making changes to be able to quantify the impact. Laury, and colleagues[11] demonstrated this approach.

SUMMARY

Moving from an M&M conference process that uses primarily a single input without expected regular outputs to one that has multiple, unbiased inputs, expected outputs, and accountability for feedback is highly complex and not easy to do. There are many challenges; the most significant of which is culture change. Success is dependent on strong leadership support, physician champion(s) in the department that are clinically respected and influencers, and collective readiness for change. For those that are successful, the experience of the authors is that the resulting changes to the patient safety culture permeates the department in many other positive ways. This new culture forms the foundational support for a meaningful PSQI curriculum, PSQI projects and other scholarly works, and incorporating PSQI topics into grand rounds presentations and journal clubs (**Fig. 3**). But most importantly, improving the care of patients.

ACKNOWLEDGMENTS

The authors would like to acknowledge several individuals at Washington University School of Medicine/Barnes-Jewish Hospital and St. Louis Children's Hospital for their enduring support of the PSQI program in the Department of Otolaryngology-Head and

Neck Surgery. These individuals include Jan Zerega, RN, Stacy Jansen, RN, Mary Taylor, JD, John Lynch, MD, and Katie Henderson, MD.

REFERENCES

1. Brennan TA, Leape LL, Laird NM, et al. Incidence of adverse events and negligence in hospitalized patients. Results of the Harvard Medical Practice Study I. N Engl J Med 1991;324:370–6.
2. Berwick DM. Continuous improvement as an ideal in health care. N Engl J Med 1989;320:53–6.
3. Chassin MR, Loeb JM. High-reliability health care: getting there from here. Milbank Q 2013;91:459–90.
4. 11 Tenets of a Safety Culture, The Joint Commission. Available at: https://www.jointcommission.org/assets/1/6/SEA_57_infographic_11_tenets_safety_culture.pdf. Accessed June 2, 2018.
5. Reason J. Human error: models and management. BMJ 2000;320:768–70.
6. Dekker S. Just culture: balancing safety and accountability. Surrey (England): Ashgate Publishing; 2007. ISBN-10: 0754672670.
7. Reason J. Managing the risks of organizational accidents. Hampshire (England): Ashgate Publishing; 1997. ISBN-10: 1840141050.
8. Dindo D, Demartines N, Clavien PA. Classification of surgical complications: a new proposal with evaluation in a cohort of 6336 patients and results of a survey. Ann Surg 2004;240:205–13.
9. Pronovost PJ, Weast B, Holzmueller CG, et al. Evaluation of the culture of safety: survey of clinicians and managers in an academic medical center. Qual Saf Health Care 2003;12:405–10.
10. AHRQ Surveys on Patient Safety Culture. Available at: https://www.ahrq.gov/sops/index.html. Accessed June 2, 2018.
11. Laury AM, Bowe SN, Lospinoso J. Integrating morbidity and mortality core competencies and quality improvement in otolaryngology. JAMA Otolaryngol Head Neck Surg 2017;143:135–40.

Resident and Fellow Engagement in Safety and Quality

Sarah N. Bowe, MD[a],*, Michael E. McCormick, MD[b,c]

KEYWORDS

- Otolaryngology • Patient safety • Quality improvement • Resident • Fellow
- Trainee • Graduate medical education • Education

KEY POINTS

- Creating a culture of safety and quality, supporting faculty development efforts, and selecting appropriate curricular resources are key steps to enhancing resident and fellow engagement.
- Developing and maintaining a "just culture" requires departmental and institutional leaders who can promote nonpunitive discussion and analysis that considers systems errors.
- House staff quality councils can serve to advise the teaching hospital on pertinent frontline issues and to engage residents directly in the improvement process.
- "Expert" educators should create and implement educational efforts and "proficient" faculty should establish cultural attitudes and norms that reflect the value of safety and quality.
- Programs must implement a dedicated curriculum including didactic education as the foundation and experiential learning opportunities as the means to reinforce key principles in practice.

Disclosure Statement: None of the authors have any commercial or financial conflicts of interest. There were no funding sources for this article. The views expressed herein are those of the authors and do not reflect the official policy or position of Brooke Army Medical Center, the US Army Medical Department, the US Army Office of the Surgeon General, the Department of the Army, the Department of Defense, or the US government.
[a] Department of Otolaryngology–Head and Neck Surgery, San Antonio Uniformed Services Health Education Consortium, 3551 Roger Brooke Drive, JBSA-Fort Sam Houston, TX 78234, USA; [b] Department of Otolaryngology and Communication Sciences, Medical College of Wisconsin, 8701 Watertown Plank Road, Milwaukee, WI 53226, USA; [c] Division of Pediatric Otolaryngology, Children's Hospital of Wisconsin, 8915 W. Connell Court, Milwaukee, WI 53226, USA
* Corresponding author.
E-mail address: DrSarahNBowe@gmail.com

INTRODUCTION

Historically, graduate medical education (GME) has focused on diagnosis and treatment; however, as health care has evolved in the era of patient safety and quality improvement (PS/QI), so has postgraduate education. In 2012, the Accreditation Council of Graduate Medical Education (ACGME) updated its approach to residency training, and for the first time, there was an explicit requirement for education in PS/QI.[1-3] Similarly, the Clinical Learning Environment Review (CLER) has created specific focuses on safety and quality in the institutional environment for trainees (residents and fellows).[4] Instruction in these principles is critical to preparing trainees for their careers after graduation, where application of PS/QI concepts will be needed for maintenance of certification and pay-for-performance reimbursement models.[5] But beyond educational and institutional requirements, there is a clear need for our trainees to learn useful PS/QI skills in order to provide better patient care in practice. Creating a culture of safety and quality, supporting faculty development efforts, and selecting appropriate curricular resources are key steps to enhancing trainee engagement in PS/QI.

FOUNDATIONS—CREATING A CULTURE OF SAFETY AND QUALITY

Successful training in PS/QI cannot be accomplished unless there exists a culture both in the department and in the organization that prioritizes safety and quality. The prime example is that of a "just culture," which involves a nonpunitive environment that fosters open and honest reporting of errors and takes systems and other nonhuman factors into consideration when investigating events.[6] In the absence of a "just culture," it can be difficult for health care providers—especially trainees—to practice free from fear of reactionary discipline when errors do occur and fear of retaliation for raising concerns about patient safety.[6] Strong interdepartmental relationships are another important ingredient to creating the desired culture, because "group culture" (which values teamwork and cohesiveness) is correlated with a strong safety climate.[7] In addition, educational programs for all types of hospital providers (eg, nurses and pharmacists) can improve communication for interdisciplinary work, helping to create and sustain a culture of safety.[8]

Because trainees from various medical and surgical specialties are often the frontline physician providers in health care, it is imperative that the GME institution and teaching hospital align their PS/QI efforts.[2] Furthermore, this alignment is mutually beneficial: GME programs can use the resources of the hospital and the hospital gains the insight and effort of engaged trainees to facilitate projects.

Many academic medical centers have capitalized on the potential that trainees have to identify safety and quality issues because of their role as frontline providers. As a result, these institutions have established house staff quality councils (HSQCs) both to advise the teaching hospital on pertinent issues and to engage residents directly in the improvement process.[9-11] More importantly, these HSQCs have provided a mechanism for direct GME-teaching hospital alignment, where representatives from both sides can strategically plan together, so that initiatives have an opportunity to reach their full potential, instead of being at odds with one another or leading to concurrent changes that obfuscate the results of the work being done.[2]

Although HSQCs are becoming more popular, they do not exist in every organization. As such, residency programs could consider eliciting a discussion with GME and hospital safety and quality leaders about creating an HSQC. Otherwise, if there is no potential to create one, most academic medical centers provide opportunities for trainees to participate as members of the distinct GME and hospital safety and quality committees.

A culture of safety and quality is an absolute necessity in order for faculty and trainees to successfully integrate PS/QI principles into practice. Efforts to align the goals and processes of the GME institution and teaching hospital, as occurs with HSQCs, can help foster a unified safety and quality mission across departments and disciplines.

FACULTY DEVELOPMENT—"EXPERT" EDUCATORS AND "PROFICIENT" FRONTLINE FACULTY

In order to fully engage trainees in the theory and practice of PS/QI, faculty must be prepared to teach these topics and reinforce them on a regular basis. The Association of American Medical Colleges (AAMC) and ACGME have made distinctions between "expert" educators who will create, implement, and evaluate education and frontline faculty who must be "proficient" in safety and quality competencies.[2] The ideal development plan must target both types of faculty.

When otolaryngology program directors were surveyed, 95% of the respondents noted that an otolaryngologist was responsible for teaching the PS/QI program.[12] Yet in 68% of those programs, the otolaryngologist responsible for instruction had not received any formal training in PS/QI methodology.[12] It is important to develop a "critical mass" of "expert" educators within each residency program.[2] However, it is first beneficial to understand the broader organizational environment. For example, some academic medical centers have sought to centralize the safety and quality education provided to a subset of "expert" educators across the teaching hospital. Two such programs include the AAMC Teaching for Quality (Te4Q) initiative and the Society of Hospital Medicine's Quality and Safety Educators Academy (QSEA).[13,14] The Te4Q initiative is a faculty development program that includes a 1.5 day, on-site workshop including an overview of adult learning principles, learner-centered education in PS/QI, and educational assessment methods.[13] Whereas, QSEA is an interactive 2.5 day, off-site program, designed to develop participants knowledge and skills in the science of PS/QI, as well as in curriculum development and assessment.[14]

If, however, the teaching hospital has not embarked on a specific curriculum for faculty development, the "expert" educators responsible for teaching PS/QI can seek out more individualized resources. One option would be to reach out to local hospital safety and quality leaders and seek recommendations for educational programs that they may have attended. Again, this helps to improve GME-teaching hospital alignment. Another option would be to engage with free, online resources that are available. In addition to a Basic Certificate in Quality and Safety, the Institute for Healthcare Improvement (IHI) also offers a course in GME Faculty Training, as well as a Massive Open Online Course (MOOC) in Practical Improvement Science in Health Care.[15,16] The GME Faculty Training consists of 6 training modules that include information about the CLER, GME and teaching hospital alignment, didactic and experiential learning facilitation, and role modeling.[15] The MOOC is a scheduled, 7-week online course focused on the principles of process improvement, including theory of change, measurable aims, and iterative, incremental tests of change.[16] Regardless of the method used, "expert" faculty development should include training in curriculum development and CLER expectations, in addition to safety and quality content, to fulfill the needs of both the training program and organization.[2]

On the other hand, the educational content to attain "proficient" frontline faculty can be similar to trainee curricula, because, at this point in time, many faculty are at the same level as trainees regarding these topics.[2] This can also establish a common PS/QI "language" for faculty and trainee communication. In the interim, frontline faculty can begin making an immediate impact on the culture of safety and quality by simply articulating the work that they are already doing in their daily practice. For example, during clinical encounters, faculty are taking time to integrate the best research with their own clinical expertise along with patient values and preferences, thus using evidence-based, patient-centered care. These are key principles of PS/QI but may be missed by trainees when not discussed explicitly.

Faculty development is essential in order to effectively teach trainees. Although "expert" educators are required to create, implement, and evaluate our PS/QI educational methods, achieving "proficient" frontline faculty is critical to establishing cultural attitudes and norms that reflect the values of safety and quality.[2]

CURRICULAR RESOURCES—DIDACTIC AND EXPERIENTIAL LEARNING

Teaching residents about safety and quality requires a dedicated curriculum. Numerous specialties have published their experiences incorporating PS/QI education into GME.[17,18] A basic foundation for an educational program in PS/QI for otolaryngology has been proposed recently.[3] This framework included quality improvement, clinical and patient safety, effective communication, systems approach to medical error, and metrics and measurement.[3] Previously successful curricula in other disciplines have combined faculty lectures with Web-based modules, including those from the World Health Organization Patient Safety (WHO PS) Curriculum Guide[19] and the IHI Open School.[20] Helpful resources that can be incorporated into a PS/QI trainee curriculum for otolaryngology are readily available from both organizations.[3]

Unfortunately, there are several obstacles that can be encountered when building a PS/QI educational program. It can be difficult to find room in an already-crowded curriculum for PS/QI topics without sacrificing more traditional lectures and surgical skills training.[3] Time and faculty expertise are common challenges as well.[3,12] Most importantly, it can be difficult to identify the most appropriate instructional methods for a particular program (ie, primarily didactic, primarily web-based, mixed didactic/web-based, etc).[3,17,18]

In general, training programs should consider 2 strategies when selecting curricular resources for PS/QI education.[2] Similar to faculty development efforts, it is first important to understand the broader organizational environment. Some hospital systems have sought to align the safety and quality experiences of trainees by implementing a core curriculum for all programs.

The San Antonio Uniformed Services Health Education Consortium (SAUSHEC) Subcommittee for PS/QI developed a Common Core Curriculum for Quality and Safety (C3QS) to address important organizational ACGME CLER requirements.[21] Incoming interns and residents complete the 7 IHI Open School Patient Safety modules[20] before the start of their training programs. This was done to establish a common PS "language" so that trainees could engage effectively in interdepartmental teams, as well as establish a clear commitment to a "culture of safety." In addition, all trainees are required to complete the entire IHI Open School Basic Certificate before residency graduation.[21] When organizational mandates exist, it is critically important to incorporate this into the training program's educational strategies. For example, the SAUSHEC Department of Otolaryngology developed and instituted a comprehensive curriculum using their organization's mandatory core requirements as a foundation. Then, faculty-led lectures were developed to reinforce the key principles from each IHI module.[22] Notably, the educators assessed their residents before and after the curriculum was implemented and found a significant increase in scores on the Quality Improvement Knowledge Application Tool – Revised. The investigators have provided full access to their comprehensive curriculum, which is available as supplemental material to their article.[22]

In contrast, some teaching hospitals have not standardized any core requirements for PS/QI education but instead have allowed each training program to customize their own curriculum.[2] For example, the Department of Otolaryngology at the Indiana University School of Medicine partnered with their local Veterans Affairs Medical Center to use the "Lean" process improvement strategy—initially originated in the manufacturing industry—as a certification program for their trainees.[23] Following implementation, several trainees achieved Yellow or Green Belt certification. In addition, numerous departmental outcomes directly attributable to the Lean training were noted, including multiple research awards, national presentations, and publications in high-impact journals.[23] As mentioned previously, another option for programs is to use and adapt the WHO PS or IHI courses to instruct their trainees in fundamental PS/QI concepts. Whatever the curriculum, programs should empower trainees to implement the learned concepts and methods and become active participants in PS/QI activities within their organizations. This "blended" approach of combining didactics with experiential learning is a proven effective adult learning model.[3,18,22]

With a proper educational framework in place, execution of PS/QI becomes natural.[3] Therefore, it is not surprising that 86% of responding otolaryngology program directors noted that a resident-driven QI project was necessary to satisfy graduation requirements.[12] When done properly, projects embody PS/QI principles in action, including the following key steps: definition of the problem, identification of key stakeholders, evidence of root cause analysis, choice of project, potential interventions, proposed intervention, and implementation and evaluation of the intervention.[24]

Although it seems that OHNS residency programs are engaged in this work, very little has been published on the topic. A recent systematic review on "Patient Safety and Quality Improvement in Otolaryngology Education" noted a complete lack of studies "translating evidence into safer care."[25] To address this gap, the investigators suggested that otolaryngology providers "look at patient data over time before, immediately after a PS/QI program was implemented, and again 6 to 12 months later to ensure that improvement is sustained." Clearly, meaningful PS/QI projects that have the potential to lead to measurable improvements in clinical process or outcome measures take time and resources. Most likely, the disconnect between trainee involvement in QI projects and the lack of publications on the topic is a result of the limited time and resources available to carry out longitudinal projects.

Thus, when considering PS/QI project work with trainees, programs may consider 3 strategies that vary depending on the ownership of the project. The first strategy involves projects that are truly trainee-driven. For example, under the current state of resident duty hour restrictions, the junior residents in one otolaryngology program were dissatisfied with the policy for assessing isolated nasal bone fractures during overnight call.[26] As a result, they worked with members of the emergency medicine and oral surgery departments to develop a mutually agreed on, evidence-based algorithm to test during overnight trauma call, planning to assess the effects on consultation rate, patient outcomes, and resident work hours.[26] However, similar to the findings noted by Gettelfinger and colleagues, there is only evidence of the initial steps of PS/QI project work, but a lack of follow-through on examining results over time. This is frequently the risk with individual trainee-driven projects as they move on to different rotations or graduate, and sustained interest in the topic by other trainees or faculty is not present. Momentum is easily lost when there are not multiple stakeholders involved in a PS/QI project.

The second strategy involves projects that are driven at the organizational level. In this approach, the project is connected to pertinent PS/QI concerns in the context of the larger health care system. As a result, there is usually greater access to resources and support. This provides an opportunity for trainees to engage in "multigenerational" projects, where they can participate in ongoing, longitudinal work, ideally for at least one full cycle of intervention selection, implementation, and evaluation.[11] The third strategy involves projects implemented at the departmental level. Similar to institutional level projects, trainees may transition the projects over time, while still maintaining the overall principles of continuous improvement.

The most integral aspect of education in PS/QI that has been noted by program directors is participation in morbidity and mortality (M&M) conferences.[3,12] The M&M conference is a long-standing tradition in surgical training programs and should be the cornerstone of PS/QI in GME. As PS/QI culture has evolved, it has been increasingly recognized that medical errors are not simply the result of human error, but rather they indicate systemic flaws, which then allow error to occur. As a result, residency programs have adapted their M&M conferences into critical evaluations of patient care episodes, many of which use the framework of the 6 ACGME competencies as their mechanism for analysis.[27,28] A similar trend has started in otolaryngology programs, where key PS/QI principles are discussed more explicitly using standardized communication tools and templates.[12,29,30] A more detailed discussion on these changes can be found in "Re-thinking Morbidity and Mortality Conference" by Brian Nussenbaum and Richard A. Chole, in this issue.

In order to effectively teach trainees about safety and quality, training programs must implement a dedicated curriculum including didactic education as the foundation. Then, experiential learning opportunities can reinforce key principles and support their integral role in providing the best patient care.

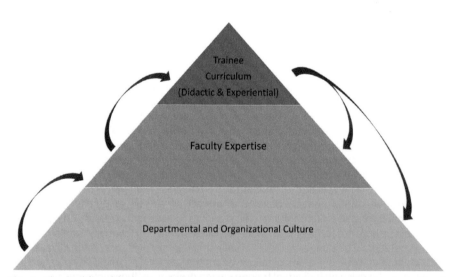

Fig. 1. The building blocks to resident and fellow engagement in safety and quality. A strong departmental and organizational culture serves as the foundation. Then, faculty and trainee education can arise. Finally, active participation in PS/QI work by both faculty and trainees will then mutually enhance the underlying culture.

SUMMARY

Developing an effective PS/QI curriculum in a training program is a daunting task but can be achieved by first focusing on the larger picture and then refining the granular details. Nurturing a culture of PS/QI within the organization and department is a foundational first step (**Fig. 1**). In doing so, programs can develop individual faculty as experts in safety and quality. When faculty has effective training in the core principles and methods, they can then implement a curriculum that is composed of both didactic and experiential learning for their trainees. With appropriate education, both faculty and trainees can become active and critical components of the organizational culture, identifying and completing meaningful projects and leading to the ultimate goal of improving the safety and quality of patient care.

REFERENCES

1. Nasca TJ, Philibert I, Brigham T, et al. The next GME accreditation system – rationale and benefits. N Engl J Med 2012;366:1051–6.
2. Tess A, Vidyarthi A, Yang J, et al. Bridging the gap: a framework and strategies for integrating the quality and safety mission of teaching hospitals and graduate medical education. Acad Med 2015;90:1251–7.
3. McCormick ME, Stadler ME, Shah RK. Embedding quality and safety in otolaryngology-head and neck surgery education. Otolaryngol Head Neck Surg 2015;152:778–82.
4. Weiss KB, Wagner R, Nasca TJ. Development, testing, and implementation of the ACGME and Clinical Learning Environment Review (CLER) program. J Grad Med Educ 2012;4:396–8.
5. Vila PM, Schneider JS, Piccirillo JF, et al. Understanding quality measures in otolaryngology – head and neck surgery. JAMA Otolaryngol Head Neck Surg 2016;142:86–90.
6. Marx D. Patient safety and the 'just culture': a primer for healthcare executives. In: Agency for Healthcare Research and Quality Patient Safety Network. 2001. Available at: www.chpso.org/sites/main/file-attachments/marx_primer.pdf. Accessed April 24, 2018.
7. Singer SJ, Falwell A, Gaba DM, et al. Identifying organizational cultures that promote patient safety. Health Care Manage Rev 2009;34:300–11.
8. Morello RT, Lowthian JA, Barker AL, et al. Strategies for improving patient safety culture in hospitals: a systematic review. BMJ Qual Saf 2013;22:11–8.
9. Fleischut PM, Faggiani SL, Evans AS, et al. The effect of a novel housestaff quality council on quality and patient safety. Jt Comm J Qual Patient Saf 2012;38:311–7.
10. Dixon JL, Papaconstantinou HT, Erwin JP, et al. House staff quality council: one institution's experience to integrate resident involvement in patient care improvement initiatives. Ochsner J 2013;13:394–9.
11. Morrison RJ, Bowe SN, Brenner MJ. Teaching quality improvement and patient safety in residency education: strategies for meaningful resident quality and safety initiatives. JAMA Otolaryngol Head Neck Surg 2017;143:1069–70.
12. Bowe SN. Quality improvement in otolaryngology residency: survey of program directors. Otolaryngol Head Neck Surg 2016;154:349–54.
13. Teaching for quality. In: Association American Medical Colleges. 2018. Available at: https://www.aamc.org/initiatives/cei/te4q/. Accessed April 22, 2018.
14. Myers JS, Tess A, Glasheen JJ. The Quality and Safety Educators Academy: fulfilling an unmet need for faculty development. Am J Med Qual 2014;29:5–12.

15. GME faculty training courses. In: Institute for Healthcare Improvement. 2018. Available at: http://www.ihi.org/education/IHIOpenSchool/Chapters/Groups/Faculty/Pages/Courses.aspx. Accessed April 22, 2018.
16. Practical improvement science in healthcare: a roadmap for getting results – A MOOC (Massive Open Online Course). In: Institute for Healthcare Improvement. 2018. Available at: http://www.ihi.org/education/WebTraining/Webinars/Practical-Improvement-Science-in-Health-Care/Pages/default.aspx. Accessed April 22, 2018.
17. Wong BM, Etchells EE, Kuper A, et al. Teaching quality improvement and patient safety to trainees: a systematic review. Acad Med 2010;85:1425–39.
18. Wong BM, Levinson W, Shojania KG. Quality improvement in medical education: current state and future directions. Med Educ 2012;46:107–9.
19. WHO Multi-professional Patient Safety Curriculum Guide. In: World Health Organization. 2018. Available at: http://www.who.int/patientsafety/education/mp_curriculum_guide/en/. Accessed April 22, 2018.
20. IHI Open School. In: Institute for Healthcare Improvement. 2018. Available at: http://www.ihi.org/education/ihiopenschool/Pages/default.aspx. Accessed April 22, 2018.
21. Nagy CJ, Zernzach RC, Jones WS, et al. Common core curriculum for quality and safety: a novel instrument for cultivating trainee engagement in quality improvement and patient safety. J Grad Med Educ 2015;7:272–4.
22. Bowe SN, Laury AM, Kepchar JJ, et al. Programmatic assessment of a comprehensive quality improvement curriculum in an otolaryngology residency. Otolaryngol Head Neck Surg 2016;155:729–32.
23. Elghouche AN, Lobo BC, Wannemuehler TJ. Lean belt certification: pathway for student, resident, and faculty development and scholarship. Otolaryngol Head Neck Surg 2016;154:785–8.
24. Leenstra JL, Beckman TJ, Reed DA. Validation of a method for assessing resident physicians' quality improvement proposals. J Gen Intern Med 2007;22:1330–4.
25. Gettelfinger JD, Paulk PB, Schmalbach CE. Patient safety and quality improvement in otolaryngology education. Otolaryngol Head Neck Surg 2017;156:991–8.
26. Lanigan A, Lospinoso J, Bowe SN, et al. The nasal fracture algorithm: a case for protocol-driven management to optimize care and resident work hours. Otolaryngol Head Neck Surg 2017;156:1041–3.
27. Rosenfeld JC. Using the morbidity and mortality conference to teach and assess the ACGME general competencies. Curr Surg 2005;62:664–9.
28. Kauffman RM, Landman MP, Shelton J, et al. The use of a multidisciplinary morbidity and mortality conference to incorporate ACGME general competencies. J Surg Educ 2011;68:303–8.
29. Laury AM, Bowe SN, Lospinoso J. Integrating morbidity and mortality core competencies and quality improvement in otolaryngology. Otolaryngol Head Neck Surg 2017;143:135–40.
30. McMullen CP, Mehta V. Integrating quality improvement into the otolaryngology morbidity and mortality conference. JAMA Otolaryngol Head Neck Surg 2017;143:140–1.

Anesthesia Safety in Otolaryngology

Andrew T. Waberski, MD[a], Alexandra G. Espinel, MD[b],
Srijaya K. Reddy, MD, MBA[c],*

KEYWORDS

- Patient safety • Anesthesia • Otolaryngologic diseases • Airway management

KEY POINTS

- Good communication and a high level of cooperation between the surgeon and anesthesiologist are imperative for otolaryngologic procedures.
- Many patients presenting for otolaryngologic surgery have multiple comorbidities that should be optimized prior to surgery.
- In addition to appreciating the anatomy and physiology of structures in the surgical field, the anesthesiologist should be able to facilitate surgery while providing adequate oxygenation, depth of anesthesia, and prompt return of consciousness and airway reflexes after surgery.
- After airway surgery, there are many risks of complications, including but not limited to, laryngospasm, bleeding, and airway obstruction.
- Intraoperative management techniques should also focus on minimizing these risks.

INTRODUCTION

Head and neck surgery integrates some of the most challenging types of cases for the anesthesiologist. Medical comorbidities, complex airways, unique surgical positioning, and need for a smooth emergence from anesthesia create a challenging paradigm for safe anesthetic management. A thorough preoperative history and physical examination of comorbidities and anatomic airway anomalies are crucial. Both the anesthesiologist and otolaryngologist share in the responsibility of safe airway

Disclosure Statement: The authors do not have any commercial or financial conflicts of interest or funding sources to disclose.
[a] Division of Anesthesiology, Pain and Perioperative Medicine, Children's National Health System, The George Washington University School of Medicine and Health Sciences, 111 Michigan Avenue Northwest, Washington, DC 20010, USA; [b] Division of Otolaryngology, Children's National Health System, The George Washington University School of Medicine and Health Sciences, 111 Michigan Avenue Northwest, Washington, DC 20010, USA; [c] Division of Pediatric Anesthesiology, Monroe Carell Jr. Children's Hospital at Vanderbilt, Vanderbilt University School of Medicine, 2200 Children's Way Suite 3116, Nashville, TN 37232, USA
* Corresponding author.
E-mail address: srijaya.k.reddy@vumc.org

Otolaryngol Clin N Am 52 (2019) 63–73
https://doi.org/10.1016/j.otc.2018.08.012
0030-6665/19/© 2018 Elsevier Inc. All rights reserved.

management and readiness for alternative airway interventions if necessary. Each patient and procedure is distinct and can differ with the type and depth of anesthetic, patient positioning, method of oxygenation and ventilation, and plan for emergence.

PREOPERATIVE ASSESSMENT

Safety in airway manipulation begins with a thorough preoperative history, physical examination, and radiographic evaluation of potential anatomic obstacles. Patients requiring head and neck surgery typically have multiple associated medical comorbidities. In the preoperative period the anesthesiologist must review cardiovascular, respiratory, endocrine, oncologic, and smoking history. Cardiovascular evaluation should include history of coronary artery disease, hypertension, cerebral vascular disease, cardiac function, exercise tolerance, and medication adherence. Patients with chronic obstructive pulmonary disease or reactive airway disease should be optimized preoperatively with bronchodilators and steroids when indicated. Plans should be made for patients requiring positive pressure support in the postoperative period, for example, patients with obstructive sleep apnea requiring continuous positive airway pressure (CPAP) or major surgery requiring prolonged intubation. Endocrine evaluation includes management of diabetic blood sugars, thyroid hormones, acromegaly airway changes, and calcium levels in the perioperative period. In the pediatric population, care must be taken to evaluate and understand the dysmorphic, metabolic, and genetic syndromes and their appropriate management.

Preoperative airway evaluation includes the history of difficult airway, airway examination, and endoscopic and imaging studies. History of airway manipulation ought to be considered with caution because the airway may become difficult over time with the progression of a disease process. Anatomic abnormalities whether from congenital, cancerous, or degenerative processes should be clearly appreciated prior to manipulation.

Radiographic images, including lateral x-rays, CT scans, MRIs, and endoscopy, can assist with oropharyngeal, laryngeal, and tracheal structural assessment. CT scans and MRIs aid in delineation of impinging masses or structures from a patent upper and lower airway. Fiberoptic nasal or oral endoscopy is particularly useful for evaluating dynamic supraglottic changes during spontaneous respiration.

ANESTHETIC SAFETY CONSIDERATIONS

For decades, anesthesiologists have advocated for patient safety. Advances in medications, airway manipulation, monitoring, and medical management have led to tremendous improvements in safety with surgery and anesthesia. The choice of anesthetic technique depends on the scope of surgical airway manipulation and patient comorbidities.

Monitoring

The standards for anesthetic monitoring are widely accepted and continuously reviewed by the American Society of Anesthesiologists (ASA) and European Board of Anaesthesiology.[1,2] These include monitors for anesthetic equipment compliance and function in addition to patient vital sign monitors. The anesthesiologist is vigilant and responsive to a patient's clinical status with or without monitor presence. Common monitoring devices for adequate oxygenation and ventilation include pulse oximetry, end-tidal carbon dioxide, airway pressure, and gas concentration measurements. Audible alarms are used for awareness and detection of potential adverse within the operating room.

Airway Management Strategy

It is crucial to patient safety that the anesthesiologist, surgeon, and perioperative staff be aware of airway management strategies for all otolaryngology procedures. Ineffective ventilation and oxygenation may have devastating outcomes for a patient. Multidisciplinary education, seasoned airway specialists, and advanced airway equipment are shown to reduce the incidence of surgical airway and morbidity.[3] Within the specialty of anesthesiology, strategies for airway management have been deliberated, published, and updated by the Task Force on Management of the Difficult Airway by the ASA and by members of the Difficult Airway Society (DAS).[4,5] Formulating a safe approach to airway management for each otolaryngology patient is crucial to providing safe anesthesia. In addition, multiple advances in airway equipment and training have elevated the practice of safe airway management. The reports from the Fourth National Audit Project (NAP4) of anesthetic airway-related deaths in the UK showed a mortality rate of 5.6 per million anesthetics.[6] Identifiable factors for airway complications in NAP4 included inadequate airway evaluation and planning, serial intubation attempts, improper utilization of equipment, inexperienced technique, and delays in assessment and treatment of airway events.[7] Skilled airway management begins with proper face mask ventilation technique, familiarity with use of supraglottic airway devices, direct laryngoscopy, fiberoptic intubation, video-assisted laryngoscopy, and the surgical airway.

Face mask ventilation

Evaluation for predictors of difficulty with face mask ventilation include BMI greater than or equal to 30 kg/m^2, presence of facial hair, Mallampati class III or IV, age greater than or equal to 57 years, limited jaw and neck mobility, and snoring.[8] The reported incidence of difficult mask ventilation in anesthetic cases is between 1% and 2% and inability to mask ventilate 0.1% and 0.2%.[8,9] Training on airway evaluation for potential difficulty with mask ventilation is imperative to limit potential hazardous scenarios of inability to ventilate. Patients with potential for difficulty with mask ventilation should be addressed with extreme caution during the anesthetic induction with preference toward the awake or spontaneous breathing patient for securing the airway. Difficulty with mask ventilation arises from an inappropriate face-mask seal or obstruction from the nasopharynx to the trachea. Strategies to assist with mask ventilation include placement of an oral or nasal airway, 2-handed mask technique, and ventilator assistance.

Supraglottic airway devices

Initially marketed as a less invasive airway technique for an uncomplicated anesthetic, the supraglottic airway device has been successfully used for airway management during cardiac arrest, in the prehospital setting, and for advanced airway techniques.[10] The supraglottic airway device functions to prop open the oropharyngeal airway and allow for unrestricted gas exchange. Because these devices are not placed within the trachea, the supraglottic airway device is not considered a secure airway from aspiration and controlled ventilation. The latest supraglottic airway devices have advanced the safety in airway management by their high success rates for insertion, ability to ventilate at high pressures, and ability to decompress the stomach with the device. Many different devices have been created, including but not limited to LMA Classic (Teleflex, Morrisville, NC), LMA Flexible (Teleflex, Morrisville, NC), LMA Fastrach (Teleflex, Morrisville, NC), air-Q (Cookgas, St. Louis, MO) self pressurizing intubating laryngeal airway, LMA ProSeal (Teleflex, Morrisville, NC), LMA Supreme (Teleflex, Morrisville, NC), and the i-gel (Intersurgical, East Syracuse, NY). Although considered an unsecure airway, the second generation of supraglottic airway devices has a separate chamber build into the device to allow for gastric decompression.[10]

The incidence of pulmonary aspiration with the first-generation LMA Classic is 2.3 per 10,000 cases.[11] Complications with the placement of a supraglottic airway device are rare. The most frequent adverse event is a postoperative sore throat commonly seen with multiple attempts at insertion, overinflation of the cuff, or prolonged surgical time.[10] Supraglottic devices have been incorporated as rescue airway devices in guidelines proposed by the Task Force on Management of the Difficult Airway by the ASA and the DAS.[4,5]

Laryngoscopy

The incidence of difficulty or failure with intubation varies by presentation and is highest in the obstetric and emergent surgical patient population. It is important to clarify the definition of difficulty with intubation with respect to the device used for laryngoscopy, manipulation techniques, and number of attempts by a skilled provider. In addition, the inability to visualize the vocal cords or pass an endotracheal tube (ETT) under laryngoscopy is an important distinction. Unsuccessful tracheal intubation ranges in incidence from 0.05% to 0.3% and cannot intubate or ventilate at less than 0.02%.[12] These published incidences do not delineate standardized laryngoscopy training, techniques, underreporting, or type of patient population. These low percentages for difficulty with intubation show the safety of airway management in modern medicine but still highlight a potential for improvement.[6]

Complications attributed to multiple attempts, defined as greater than 2 attempts, at airway management include hypoxia, aspiration, bradycardia, and cardiac arrest.[13] Limiting repeated attempts at intubation to 2 or fewer is supported in the ASA and DAS guidelines for difficult airway management.[4,5]

Fiberoptic intubation

Patients presenting with limited mouth opening, intraoral obstruction, and limited or restricted cervical mobility benefit from fiberoptic intubation. The fiberoptic scope is a semirigid device that can be maneuvered under indirect visualization, through narrow airway openings. This method prevents highly stimulated anatomic distortion, as with laryngoscopy, and, therefore, is used with great success in the awake or sedated patient with a known difficult airway.[14] Fiberoptic intubation also serves as a rescue device, but time to successful intubation is typically prolonged by technique, experience, and low operator frequency.[15]

Video-assisted laryngoscopy

The advent of the video-assisted laryngoscope has revolutionized the practice of difficult airway management. Video laryngoscopy techniques have become common practice and are detailed in society guidelines of difficult airway management. These devices allow for superior indirect visualization of the glottis and placement of endotracheal tube.[16] Furthermore, Cochrane database analysis of more than 60 studies shows a significant difference of fewer failed intubations, including those with anticipated difficult airways, compared with direct laryngoscopy.[17]

Surgical airway

If and when endotracheal intubation cannot be achieved by the modalities discussed previously, a surgical airway may be indicated. Transtracheal needle ventilation, percutaneous tracheostomy, or open tracheostomy in the operating room should be performed by the otolaryngologist in collaboration with the anesthesiologist.[18] Potential intraoperative complications of tracheostomy include cuff perforation, loss of airway, difficulty with tracheostomy tube insertion, and airway fire.[19]

Positioning

Because otolaryngologists and anesthesiologists work together to secure and maintain the airway during surgery, ideal positioning with unobstructed access to the airway is a serious safety concern. Prior to induction of anesthesia, it is essential for both teams to discuss the optimal placement and method for securing the ETT, patient positioning, and acknowledging the possibility of an unplanned extubation.

Determining where the head of the operating table will be for the surgery allows the anesthesiologist to plan for turning the bed and positioning lines and circuits such that dislodgement of the ETT is minimized. Care must be taken when moving the bed, and it is recommended that the ETT and circuit be temporarily disconnected while turning. After reconnecting, appropriate ventilation and oxygenation should again be confirmed.

Because most otolaryngologic procedures involve turning the head, repositioning the neck, access to the oral cavity, and ETT manipulation, the risk for unplanned extubation is high. Communication prior to patient repositioning and ETT manipulation is essential so that the anesthesiologist can be prepared for and assist in ensuring the ETT remains in the correct position. Additionally, the anesthesiologist must rely on close monitoring of end-tidal CO_2, ventilation, and oxygenation, because slight changes can be the first sign of accidental extubation during the procedure.

Despite these precautions, inadvertent extubation can still occur. Throughout the duration of the case, the anesthesiologist must be prepared to re-establish the airway emergently. This includes having necessary medications and equipment readily available. It must also be kept in mind that re-establishing the airway after unplanned extubation can be more difficult than the initial intubation. Factors, such as airway edema, secretions, and intraoperative patient positioning, may prevent the best visualization of the larynx.

Maintenance of Anesthesia

The depth of anesthesia depends on the surgical case and patient safety. Typical general anesthetic maintenance is provided through a combination of inhalational and intravenous medications. Inhalational anesthetics work in 2 parts: to inhibit spinal cord reflexes to noxious stimuli and to depress consciousness at the cortical level.[20] Side effects of inhaled anesthetics include agitation with induction and emergence, postoperative nausea and vomiting (PONV), and decrease in systemic vascular resistance and cardiac output. Intravenous benzodiazepines and opioids minimize the higher concentration requirements of inhaled anesthetics. Additionally, muscle relaxants also decrease the inhaled anesthetic concentration. This balanced anesthetic technique provides a more comfortable transition to emergence and the postoperative period. Total intravenous anesthetic provides a reliable depth of anesthesia when maintenance with inhalational anesthetics are interrupted, such as during bronchoscopy procedures. The choice of anesthetic agent is dependent on surgical procedure and patient comorbidities.

Opioid medications provide significant analgesic and sedative properties while maintaining hemodynamic stability. Typical side effects of opioids include respiratory depression, PONV, and decreases in heart rate.[21,22] Synthetic opioids differ from each other in their potency, onset, duration, and half-life. Typically, short-acting opioids are administered during the perioperative period for quick titration and shortened emergence. Caution should be exercised in those patients who have concomitant respiratory insufficiency (eg, chronic obstructive pulmonary disease) or airway obstruction (eg, sleep apnea and tumors). Administration of opioids to these patients could exacerbate hypoxia, hypercarbia, and lead to respiratory arrest.

Ventilation and Oxygenation Strategies

Spontaneous ventilation can be maintained for procedures that require continuous or intermittent airway manipulation. Preventing patient movement in this situation is best achieved with a combination of intravenous and inhalation medications that allow for adequate depth of anesthesia and analgesia while maintaining adequate unobstructed respiratory mechanics. Intravenous anesthetics, such as dexmedetomidine, propofol, and ketamine, blunt airway reflexes while maintaining spontaneous ventilation.

Additional shared airway techniques include jet ventilation and intermittent apneic ventilation. Jet ventilation is manual administration of intratracheal high-pressure oxygen regulated by time to allow for exhalation. This technique can be used for bronchoscopic and lanygoscopic surgical techniques in addition to a rescue airway oxygenation strategy. Jet ventilation is typically reserved for specific cases for the high incidence of complications, including barotrauma.[23] Both shared airway methods require constant communication between the otolaryngologist and anesthesiologist in providing safe and efficient procedural care.

Airway Fire Prevention

Airway fires occur at an alarming rate and have been the subject of many anesthesia closed claims. The main causes of airway fires and burns are supplemental oxygen in poorly ventilated surgical fields and the presence of combustible solutions or fabrics, both typically ignited by cautery.

Prevention of airway fires is the responsibility of all operating room staff to ensure that the patient is receiving the least harmful concentration of oxygen at the safest setting. Steps should be taken to limit leakage and trapping of high concentrations of oxygen in close proximity to the patient. Additionally, skin preparation solutions should be allowed sufficient time to dry, and gauze and sponges used during surgery should be wet to prevent combustion.[24] This can be accomplished by the use of a secure airway with a properly functioning cuffed ETT and, when clinically appropriate, minimizing oxygen concentrations to less than 50%.[25] In addition, proper ventilation and scavenging of expired and leaking oxygen help prevent airway fires.[24]

The ASA Task Force on Operating Room Fires advises all staff to undergo education on operating room fire safety, perform fire safety drills, and adequately prepare for management of fires. Consensus on the management of an airway fire includes stopping the flow of oxygen, removal of flammable agents (eg, ETT and surgical drapes), extinguishing the fire with saline, and securing the patient's airway.[24]

Management of Postoperative Nausea and Vomiting

PONV occurs with high frequency and can increase length of stay. Contributing factors that increase the risk of PONV include length of anesthetic, use of volatile anesthetics, administration of opioids, and history of motion sickness.[26] Several different classifications of medications are typically administered in the perioperative period to prevent and treat PONV; these include steroids, serotonin inhibitors, promotility agents, antihistaminergic agents, and anticholinergics.

Emergence from Anesthesia and Criteria for Extubation

Smooth emergence from the anesthetized state is crucial to patient safety and comfort. Irritation from an airway device, seen to a larger extent with endotracheal tubes, causes a reflex coughing response that can have significant hemodynamic perturbations. Coughing and straining with emergence or in the postoperative period have been shown to increase the risk of hematoma or hemorrhage in neck surgery.[27] Early implementation of intravenous analgesics and anesthetics helps prevent the typical aggressive and agitated state of emergence from anesthesia. Both dexmedetomidine and remifentanil have also shown to help with smooth emergence.

For complete emergence and resumption of unassisted spontaneous ventilation, the patient should have an unobstructed airway, with adequate laryngeal muscle tone to prevent aspiration, and adequate ventilator function. Evaluation for extubation begins with minimizing postoperative risk for hypoxia, hypercarbia, bleeding, surgical outcome, and airway obstruction.

Residual neuromuscular blockage and hypotonic pathology prevent adequate ventilation and may incite upper airway obstruction. Standard neuromuscular reversal occurs with acetylcholinesterase antagonists that increase the available acetylcholine at the neuromuscular junction for adequate muscular strength prior to extubation; a new medication, sugammadex, has proved superior in decreasing residual muscle weakness without the typical cholinergic side effects.[28]

Endotracheal extubation can be performed in the well-anesthetized patient prior to emergence, described as "deep extubation." This technique can be safely used in pediatric anesthesia in an effort to minimize agitation and coughing.[29] Additionally, the use of an laryngeal mask airway significantly decreases the risk of laryngospasm, coughing, and hoarse voice that can occur with emergence.[30]

POSTOPERATIVE SAFETY CONSIDERATIONS
Airway Obstruction

After otolaryngology procedures, patients are at a high risk for postoperative airway obstruction. Given the anatomy and extent of the surgery performed, airway obstruction can be due to airway edema, upper airway obstruction, vocal cord paresis, or increased secretions. These can be manifested by apnea, stridor, hoarseness, or drooling. Prior to extubation, the anesthesiologist and surgeon should discuss optimal timing for extubation as well as the potential sites and causes for postoperative obstruction.

Edema anywhere from the nasopharynx to glottis can contribute to postoperative airway obstruction. The location of the surgery determines the location of the associated edema and site of obstruction. In the upper airway, this can often be bypassed and managed with the use of a nasal or oral airway. Edema that is present at the supraglottis or below, however, may necessitate reintubation. It is important to recall that this edema may make reintubation more difficult; thus, these patients should be approached as would a difficult airway.

Patients undergoing surgery for obstructive sleep apnea are especially at risk for airway obstruction postoperatively. Risk factors increasing the likelihood of this include increased body mass index and apnea-hypopnea index.[31] Patients should be monitored for oxygen desaturation and apnea in the postanesthesia recovery unit, with inpatient observation for those high-risk patients. CPAP be may be used if not contraindicated by the surgery.

Stridor or hoarseness in the postoperative period may be related to airway edema; however, it can also be a sign of bilateral or unilateral vocal cord paresis. Vocal cord paresis can be secondary to injury of the recurrent laryngeal nerve intraoperatively or due to pressure of the ETT cuff on the anterior branches of the nerve.[32] Unilateral cord paresis also can be observed; however, bilateral vocal cord immobility may be life threatening for some patients. In a stable patient, vocal cord motion can be assessed via flexible laryngoscopy. Patients with bilateral cord immobility typically demonstrate signs of upper airway obstruction and oxygen desaturation.[33]

The nature of many head and neck procedures results in increased oral secretions postoperatively. This is due to both increased salivary production and a less efficient swallow mechanism due to surgery. Patients may cough or drool and are best managed sitting upright with a suction device to assist in clearing their secretions. Patients may be required to be nothing by mouth, with nasogastric tube placement until they can sufficiently clear their secretions.[34]

In addition to airway obstruction, patients are at risk for progressive respiratory failure. Major contributing factors are perioperative opioids and benzodiazepines that increase the risk of sedation, upper airway obstruction, and hypopnea. This is especially true for patients with diagnosed obstructive sleep apnea, because they have an increased sensitivity to opioids and worsening postoperative respiratory dynamic due to central sleep apnea or airway obstruction.[35] Practice guidelines for anesthetic management of patients with obstructive sleep apnea include awake extubation, minimizing opioids, performing regional analgesic techniques, administering supplemental oxygen and positive pressure, and inserting supraglottic airway devices when appropriate.[36] Other contributing factors to postoperative airway obstruction include stridor, hoarseness, secretions, and airway edema. In these cases, administration of steroids, supplemental oxygen with heliox, and racemic epinephrine may be appropriate.

Bleeding

Routine postoperative care requires that a patient's surgical site has adequate hemostasis. Because many surgical sites are directly continuous with the airway, postoperative bleeding can quickly cause an airway emergency as blood is obstructing the airway. Postoperative bleeding may occur up to 2 weeks after surgery. It can initially present with a sentinel bleed that appears minor and to self-resolve followed by a larger amount of bleeding.[37] In most instances, the airway must be secured prior to controlling the bleeding. Airway management is thus complicated by the bleeding, obstructing airway visualization. In cases of hemorrhage present, patients should have adequate volume resuscitation and be typed and cross-matched for blood product administration and advanced airway precautions due to risk of aspiration and difficulty with intubation should be undertaken.

Bleeding in sites not directly connected to the airway can manifest as a neck hematoma. The hematoma can cause mass effect on the surrounding neck structures resulting in airway compromise. Hematoma evacuation immediately relieves the mass effect; however, laryngeal edema persists due to venous congestion from the mass effect.[38] The anesthesiologist needs to be prepared to encounter this edema when reintubating the patient.

Laryngospasm

Laryngospasm is a vagally mediated reflex closure of the vocal cords. This sudden airway obstruction can be elicited by hypocalcemia, inadequate depth of anesthesia, and stimulation from a foreign body. Although there is no widely accepted guideline for the management of laryngospasm, typical treatment to airway obstruction begins with applying 100% Fio_2 with CPAP and opening the upper airway. Ability to ventilate can be readily assessed with chest rise, end-tidal CO_2, and oxygen saturation. Complete laryngospasm can be further treated with the administration of short-acting muscle relaxants and deepening the anesthetic with intravenous medications.[39] Intubation may be difficult but appropriate to stabilize patient.

Complete airway obstruction in the spontaneously ventilated patient has the potential to cause not only hypoxia and cardiopulmonary arrest but also negative pressure pulmonary edema (NPPE). NPPE develops from elevated negative inspiratory pressure and hydrostatic pressure forcing fluid into the alveoli. Timely relief of airway obstruction is the primary step to normalizing hydrostatic pressure and redistributing intra-alveolar fluid and typically resolves within a day.[40] Mechanical ventilation and diuretic therapy are standard ICU strategies for the management of NPPE.

SUMMARY

One of the greatest advances in surgery and medicine is anesthesia. For approximately 2 centuries the practice of anesthesia has allowed for surgical procedures to be performed safely along with both patient and surgeon confidence. The favorable pharmacodynamics profiles of modern anesthetics and analgesics make their administration universally applicable to large varieties of patient populations and conditions. Additionally, technologic advances in the anesthesia workstation, ventilator, airway techniques, and airway devices provide immeasurable safety nets to patients, which are even more paramount in otolaryngologic surgery.

REFERENCES

1. Standards for basic anesthetic monitoring. Committee of origin: standards and practice parameters (approved by the ASA House of Delegates on October 21, 1986, last amended on October 20, 2010, and last affirmed on October 28, 2016). Available at: https://www.asahq.org/~media/Sites/ASAHQ/Files/Public/Resources/standards-guidelines/standards-for-basic-anesthetic-monitoring.pdf. Accessed May 6, 2016.
2. European Board of Anaesthesiology (EBA), UEMS anaesthesiology section. Recommendations for minimal monitoring during anaesthesia and recovery 2012. Available at: http://www.eba-uems.eu/resources/PDFS/safety-guidelines/EBA-Minimal-monitor.pdf. Accessed May 6, 2016.
3. Berkow LC, Greenberg RS, Kan KH, et al. Need for emergency surgical airway reduced by a comprehensive difficult airway program. Anesth Analg 2009; 109(6):1860–9.
4. Apfelbaum JL, Hagberg CA, Caplan RA, et al, American Society of Anesthesiologists Task Force on Management of the Difficult Airway. Practice guidelines for management of the difficult airway: an updated report by the American Society of Anesthesiologists Task Force on Management of the Difficult Airway. Anesthesiology 2013;118(2):251–70.
5. Frerk C, Mitchell VS, McNarry AF, et al. Difficult Airway Society intubation guidelines working group. Difficult Airway Society 2015 guidelines for management of the unanticipated difficult intubation in adults. Br J Anaesth 2015;115(6):827–48.
6. Cook TM, Woodall N, Harper J, et al, Fourth National Audit Project. Major complications of airway management in the UK: results of the Fourth National Audit Project of the Royal College of Anaesthetists and Difficult Airway Society. Part 2: intensive care and emergency departments. Br J Anaesth 2011;106(5):632–42.
7. Cook TM. Strategies for the prevention of airway complications – a narrative review. Anaesthesia 2018;73(1):93–111.
8. Kheterpal S, Han R, Tremper KK, et al. Incidence and predictors of difficult and impossible mask ventilation. Anesthesiology 2006;105(5):885–91.
9. Han R, Tremper KK, Kheterpal S, et al. Grading scalre for mask ventilation. Anesthesiology 2004;101(1):267.

10. Michalek P, Donaldson W, Vobrubova E, et al. Complications associated with the use of supraglottic airway devices in perioperative medicine. Biomed Res Int 2015;2015:746560.

11. Brimacombe JR, Berry A. The incidence of aspiration associated with the laryngeal mask airway: a meta-analysis of published literature. J Clin Anesth 1995; 7(4):297–305.

12. Rose DK, Cohen MM. The airway: problems and predictions in 18,500 patients. Can J Anaesth 1994;41(5 Pt 1):372–83.

13. Mort TC. Emergency tracheal intubation: complications associated with repeated laryngoscopic attempts. Anesth Analg 2004;99(2):607–13.

14. Weiss YG, Deutschman CS. The role of fiberoptic bronchoscopy in airway management of the critically Ill patient. Crit Care Clin 2000;16(3):445–51.

15. Yumul R, Elvir-Lazo OL, White PF, et al. Comparison of the C-MAC video laryngoscope to a flexible fiberoptic scope for intubation with cervical spine immobilization. J Clin Anesth 2016;31:46–52.

16. De Jong A, Molinari N, Conseil M, et al. Video laryngoscopy versus direct laryngoscopy for orotracheal Intubation in the intensive care unit: a systematic review and meta-analysis. Intensive Care Med 2014;40(5):629–39.

17. Lewis SR, Butler AR, Parker J, et al. Videolaryngoscopy versus direct laryngoscopy for adult patients requiring tracheal intubation. Cochrane Database Syst Rev 2016;(11):CD011136.

18. Panda N, Donahue DM. Acute airway management. Ann Cardiothorac Surg 2018; 7(2):266–72.

19. McRae K. Anesthesia for airway surgery. Anesthesiol Clin North America 2001; 19(3):497–541.

20. Perouansky M, Pearce RA, Hemmings HC. Inhaled anesthetics: mechanism of action. In: Miller RD, Cohen NH, Eriksson LI, et al, editors. Miller's anesthesia. 8th edition. Philadelphia: Saunders; 2015. p. 614–37.

21. Bailey PL, Fung MC, Price RL, et al. Differences in magnitude and duration of opioid-Induced respiratory depression and analgesia with fentanyl and sufentanil. Anesth Analg 1990;70(1):8–15.

22. Kazihiko F. Opioid analgesics. In: Miller RD, Cohen NH, Eriksson LI, et al, editors. Miller's anesthesia. 8th edition. Philadelphia: Saunders; 2015. p. 864–914.

23. Duggan LV, Ballantyne Scott B, Law JA, et al. Transtracheal jet ventilation in the 'can't intubate can't oxygenate' emergency: a systematic review. Br J Anaesth 2016;117(Suppl 1):i28–38.

24. Apfelbaum JL, Caplan RA, Barker SJ, et al, American Society of Anestthesiologists Task Force on Operating Room Fires. Practice advisory for the prevention and management of operating room fires: an updated report by the American Society of Anesthesiologists Task Force on Operating Room Fires. Anesthesiology 2013;118(2):271–90.

25. Akhtar N, Ansar F, Baig MS, et al. Airway fires during surgery: management and prevention. J Anaesthesiol Clin Pharmacol 2016;32(1):109–11.

26. Gan TJ, Diemunsch P, Habib AS, et al, Society for Ambulatory Anesthesia. Consensus guidelines for the management of postoperative nausea and vomiting. Anesth Analg 2014;118(1):85–113.

27. Lee HS, Lee BJ, Kim SW, et al. Patterns of post-thyroidectomy hemorrhage. Clin Exp Otorhinolaryngol 2009;2(2):72–7.

28. Hristovska AM, Duch P, Allingstrup M, et al. Efficacy and safety of sugammadex versus neostigmine in reversing neuromuscular blockade in adults. Cochrane Database Syst Rev 2017;(8):CD012763.

29. Valley RD, Freid EB, Bailey AG, et al. Tracheal extubation of deeply anesthetized pediatric patients: a comparison of desflurane and sevoflurane. Anesth Analg 2003;96(5):1320–4.
30. Yu SH, Beirne OR. Laryngeal mask airways have a lower risk of airway complications compared with endotracheal intubation: a systematic review. J Oral Maxillofac Surg 2010;68(10):2359–76.
31. Kandasamy T, Wright ED, Fuller J, et al. The incidence of early post-operative complications following uvulopalatopharyngoplasty: identification of predictive risk factors. J Otolaryngol Head Neck Surg 2013;42(1):15.
32. Tekin M, Acar GO, Kaytac A, et al. Bilateral vocal cord paralysis secondary to head and neck surgery. J Craniofac Surg 2012;23(1):135–7.
33. Hillel AD, Benninger M, Blitzer A, et al. Evaluation and management of bilateral vocal cord immobility. Otolaryngol Head Neck Surg 1999;121(6):760–5.
34. Wang Y, Li X, Pan Z. Analyses of functional and oncologic outcomes following supracricoid partial laryngectomy. Eur Arch Otorhinolaryngol 2015;272(11): 3463–8.
35. Brown KA, Laferriere A, Lakheeram I, et al. Recurrent hypoxemia in children is associated with increased analgesic sensitivity to opiates. Anesthesiology 2006;105(4):665–9.
36. American Society of Anesthesiologists Task Force on Perioperative Management of patients with obstructive sleep apnea. Practice guidelines for the perioperative management of patients with obstructive sleep apnea: an updated report by the American Society of Anesthesiologists Task Force on Perioperative Management of patients with obstructive sleep apnea. Anesthesiology 2014;120(2):268–86.
37. Pynnonen MA, Gillespie MB, Roman B, et al. Clinical practice guideline: evaluation of the neck mass in adults. Otolaryngol Head Neck Surg 2017;157(2_suppl): S1–30.
38. Margolick J, Wiseman SM. Risk of major complications following thyroidectomy and parathyroidectomy: utility of the NSQIP surgical risk calculator. Am J Surg 2018;215(5):936–41.
39. Hampson-Evans D, Morgan P, Farrar M. Pediatric laryngospasm. Paediatr Anaesth 2008;18(4):303–7.
40. Bhattacharya M, Kallet RH, Ware LB, et al. Negative-pressure pulmonary edema. Chest 2016;150(4):927–33.

Patient Safety in Audiology

Tommie L. Robinson Jr, PhD, CCC-SLP, FASHA, FNAP[a],*,
Tracey Ambrose, AuD, CCC-A[b], Lyuba Gitman, MD[c],
Lemmietta G. McNeilly, PhD, CCC-SLP,[d]

KEYWORDS

- Patient safety • Audiology • Medical errors • Diagnostic errors

KEY POINTS

- Patient safety issues exist in audiology, although the impact may not lead to immediately obvious adverse health care events.
- The areas of communication, patient safety education, technology, electronic health records, heath literacy, and evidence-based practice all play a role in patient safety.
- Enhanced knowledge and skills in the areas related to clinical practice and service delivery can maximize patient safety.

INTRODUCTION

Although the issue of patient safety has been studied from a medical standpoint, allied health professionals in general and communication sciences and disorders professionals specifically have not focused on this topic. This article focuses on patient safety with audiologists and their clinical practice. Although the majority of audiologists' services do not lead to adverse health care events, there are some practice areas where misdiagnoses or inappropriate treatment approaches can lead to less than adequate quality of life for the individuals served. In addition, there are areas that should be reported, analyzed, and prevented because they relate to patient safety. Several error types are reported in clinical settings, including communication, patient safety education, technology, electronic health records, health literacy, and evidence-based practice. Continuous quality-improvement programs include safety

Disclosure Statement: The authors have no financial disclosures.
[a] Division of Hearing and Speech, Children's National Health System, Scottish Rite Center for Childhood Language Disorders, George Washington University School of Medicine and Health Sciences, 111 Michigan Avenue Northwest, Washington, DC 20010, USA; [b] Division of Hearing and Speech, Children's National Health System, 111 Michigan Avenue Northwest, Washington, DC 20010, USA; [c] Division of ENT, Children's National Health System, George Washington University School of Medicine and Health Sciences, 111 Michigan Avenue Northwest, Washington, DC 20010, USA; [d] American Speech-Language-Hearing Association, 2200 Research Boulevard, Rockville, MD 20850, USA
* Corresponding author.
E-mail address: trobinso@childrensnational.org

initiatives that are essential components for organizational frameworks that result in creating a culture of patient safety.

THE DIAGNOSTIC PROCESS IS COMPLEX

Fig. 1 depicts the perspective of all participants in the diagnostic process (patient, clinician, and institutional variables) and highlights issues and the necessary skills needed to complete the diagnostic process to enhance patient safety. Essentially, each touch-point or transition of care/information is a potential point of introduction of medical error.

Patient

A patient brings a variety of considerations to the clinical operations. Patients often come to the clinical environment with little or no information regarding the stages of a disorder or its etiology or without knowing that hearing is associated with other diagnoses. Audiologists provide information and need to apply health literacy strategies when communicating with the patient. Some patients are unaware of any factors regarding their diagnosis. They need to be educated and trained to minimize impact and reduce patient safety error.

Clinician/Audiologist

Audiologists need to be competent to assess the type and severity of hearing loss and make specific recommendations and use strategies for which evidence supports targeted outcomes for treating the hearing loss. Clinicians are competent when they consider evidence regarding clinical disorders and exposure to drugs and other environmental toxins that may result in hearing loss. Audiologists should practice at the top of their license, engaging in the specific activities that require their unique knowledge, skills, and expertise. The clinician brings a variety of experiences to the clinical environment that aid in completing the diagnostic process.

It is important that audiologists clearly understand policies and procedures for accessing and maintaining patient information. Clinicians' ability to effectively solve

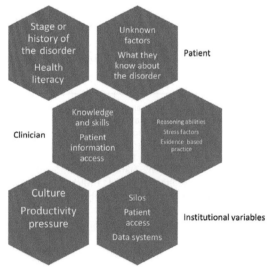

Fig. 1. Diagnosis is difficult.

problems and demonstrate emotional intelligence as they maintain resilience is important. Audiologists need to communicate clearly and use multiple methods to communicate with patients from diverse cultures. It is important for organizations to use audiologists with cultural competence to meet the needs of patients from a variety of cultures; 82.9% of audiologists working in hospitals feel qualified to address cultural and linguistic influences on service delivery and outcomes.[1]

Institutional Variables

The institution has responsibility for establishing a culture of patient safety that includes support for health professionals, strategies for maintaining health and well-being, and managing stress. Working within silos limits access to information across all of the service providers. An electronic health record that includes patient data and is accessible and used by all appropriate clinicians working with patients is important to facilitating an environment that fosters and enhances patient safety. The institution should continuously monitor the data within the system and, when an error occurs, make systemic changes to reduce the likelihood of the error being repeated by other clinicians.

SYSTEMS ERRORS

Table 1 depicts systems errors that have an impact on patient safety. The errors are divided into 3 categories: institutional, electronic, and local.

Institutional

Low staff morale increases the likelihood that errors are made. Although the data for morale overall are good in audiology, that does not negate the fact that in some institutions that may not be the case. Audiologists who own their private practices report significantly higher job satisfaction than those working in hospitals, physician offices, or public schools.[2] When morale is low, it increases the likelihood that an error is made relative to a diagnosis or other clinical encounters. The health care setting is the primary first employment setting among recent graduates; thus, it is essential that institutions provide professional development opportunities for audiologists and other health professionals.[1,2] Ongoing activities are important to enhance staff morale. Institutions must focus on these types of activities to maximize the potential of audiologists and decrease stress on professionals.

It is important for institutions to prioritize establishing a culture of patient safety. When audiologists are experiencing or working in a culture that is not conducive to the safety of patients, it increases the likelihood that safety errors are reported. Institutions are to maintain a culture that allows individuals to report issues surrounding patient safety. It is also helpful when an institution works to reduce and prevent patient safety errors.

Institutions often provide learning opportunities for professional staff with limited focus on the topic of patient safety. Audiology divisions should adopt the culture of

Table 1 Systems errors		
Institutional	**Electronic**	**Local**
• Low staff morale	• Inadequate electronic health record	• Communication breakdown
• Sick culture	• Inadequate equipment	• Clinical processes
• Limited education and training opportunities	• Failure to use equipment adequately	• Outdated policies and procedures
• Lack of response to quality-improvement data		

the institution and use it as an avenue for increased education and training in patient safety. When there is limited education and training, there is an increased likelihood that a patient safety is made.

Institutions can also make errors by having an environment that lacks responses to quality improvement. It is important to conduct continuous quality-improvement surveys and to use the data wisely to enhance service delivery. Improved use of quality-improvement data also facilitates ongoing assessment of clinical practice to reduce the number of errors associated with the clinical environment.

Electronic

"Electronic health record" as a systems error occurs when there is not an adequate reporting mechanism to allow the audiologist to see a patient's entire medical history. The electronic health record should be open so that when audiologists are evaluating a patient they can get a full view of the patient's health and medical histories. It is important to know this to be a good diagnostician. Failure may result in data that are not accurate to support an appropriate diagnosis.

"Inadequate equipment" is another systems error. When the equipment is not calibrated appropriately or not adequate to support a full-scale assessment of a patient's hearing, the result may be a patient safety issue.

Health system errors also can occur when there is adequate equipment; however, the audiologist does not know how to use it or interpret the results appropriately. This can result in patient safety errors that are rooted in misdiagnoses and maltreatments.

Local

Communication breakdowns can lead to patient safety errors on several levels in audiology. There can be communication breakdowns between the patient and the audiologist; breakdown between the audiologist and an otolaryngologist; and/or a breakdown between an audiologist and another audiologist or colleague involved in a patient's care. This can result in an adverse decision that might have an impact on the hearing of a patient.

Clinical processes are also a system error. The audiologist is responsible for providing the best clinical services using current clinical pathways and evidence-based practices. An error occurs when the audiologist does not use the appropriate process, which could lead to a miss diagnosis.

Policies and procedures errors occur when the policies and procedures are outdated and do not use current best practices. The audiologist should be on top of creating an environment where policies and procedures are updated on a regular basis. This eliminates the likelihood that an error occurs and puts in place a mechanism to combat the issue in the future.

HUMAN FACTORS

Fig. 2 depicts how the human factor plays a role in patient safety. The issues of ethics, communication, cognition, mindfulness and stress, and job satisfaction and recognition are discussed.

Ethics

Ethics is strategically place at the center of all clinical encounters. Audiologists must be aware of that all clinical decisions should be ethical in nature and there are no shortcuts.

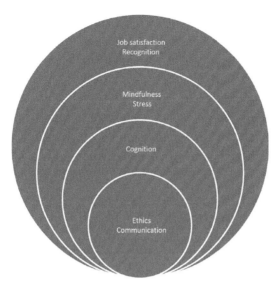

Fig. 2. Human factors. EHR, electronic health record.

Communication

Communication is also at the core of human factors that have an impact on patient safety.[3] Communication should be appropriate for every clinical encounter and that includes those from culturally and linguistically diverse populations. The communications process is important for reducing errors. When the communication process is appropriate and strong, the likelihood of an error occurring is greatly reduced.

Cognition

Cognition is at the center of several issues relative to the audiologist providing clinical services. As a part of this process, the audiologist should be able to problem solve appropriately to the situation and the clinical encounter. The audiologist should use the correct fund of knowledge to enhance the clinical encounter. Also, the audiologist's emotional intelligence should be an overarching factor.

Mindfulness and Stress

Mindfulness and stress are factors that influence patient safety. When stress is increased, it is likely that the audiologist makes a mistake in practice. Mindfulness should be at the forefront of the person, the audiologist. This aids in reducing stress and allows for the audiologist to give undivided attention to the clinical encounter and reduce the likelihood of making an error.

Job Satisfaction and Recognition

Lastly, job satisfaction and performance recognition are the final rungs associated with this figure. If all the other factors are in place, it is likely that the audiologist is satisfied that job performance and actions are being recognized, which serves as a final reward to the audiologist. This leads to the audiologist being valued by the supervisor and institution and as a result patient errors are greatly reduced.

CLINICAL APPLICATION

The cross-check principle is a widely known and taught principle in pediatric audi-ology.[4,5] Failure to use this principle continues to be seen, which negatively affects pe-diatric patients and is a patient safety issue when not used. Cross-check was originally defined as "the results of a single test are cross-checked by an independent test mea-sure."[4] Recently, it was further indicated that "...no auditory test result should be accepted and used in the diagnosis of hearing loss until it is confirmed or cross-checked by one or more independent measures. Exclusive reliance on only one or two tests, even objective auditory measures, may result in an auditory diagnosis that is, not clear or perhaps incorrect."[4] The following case examples illustrate the importance of the cross-check principle and the detrimental effects to patients when they are not used properly.

EXAMPLE 1: NEWBORN HEARING SCREENING
Clinical History

Baby boy was born full term via vaginal delivery weighing 7 lb, 10 oz. Mother received prenatal care. There were no infections or complications during pregnancy. There was no exposure to cigarettes, drugs, alcohol, or medications. There were no postbirth complications.

Audiological Testing

Baby boy failed the initial newborn hearing screening AABR and hospital follow-up screen 2 weeks later, bilaterally. At that time, he was referred to audiology clinic for follow-up testing. Hearing screen completed in audiology clinic was transient evoked otoacoustic emissions (OAEs) testing, which he passed for each ear individually and was discharged (**Table 2**).

Table 2				
Newborn hearing screen results				
Date	**Screen**	**Ear**	**Results**	**Test Type**
8/20/2015	Birth	L	Refer	AABR
8/20/2015	Birth	R	Refer	AABR
8/31/2015	Birth	L	Refer	AABR
8/31/2015	Birth	R	Refer	AABR
9/11/2015	Outpatient	R	Refer	AABR
9/11/2015	Outpatient	L	Refer	AABR
10/15/2015	Outpatient	R	Pass	OAE
10/15/2015	Outpatient	L	Pass	OAE

Abbreviatiations: L, left; R, right.

Referral

Parents express concerns about hearing ability because he does not respond consis-tently to his name/simple commands. Pediatrician referred for services, and speech and language skills were below expectations.

No reliable behavioral results were obtained at the evaluation. Immittance was consistent with normal tympanic membrane mobility and absent ipsilateral acoustic reflex screening in both ears. Distortion product OAEs (DPOAEs) were present in both ears (**Fig. 3**). Re-evaluation was consistent with initial evaluation (**Fig. 4**).

Audiogram at 16 mo

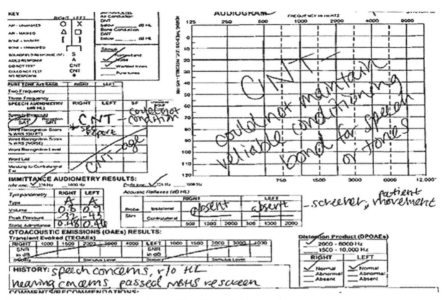

Fig. 3. Audiogram depicting inconsistent/unreliable results.

Repeat audiogram and DPOAEs (17 mo):

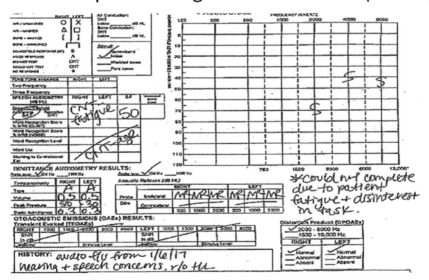

Fig. 4. Repeat audiogram 1 month after initial.

Auditory brainstem response testing was completed at (18 months)
Click stimulus Right ear: rarefaction and condensation polarities were used at 80 dB for normal hearing level (nHL) and at 90 dB nHL (**Fig. 5**). Reversal of cochlear microphonic—with no measurable neural waveform present.

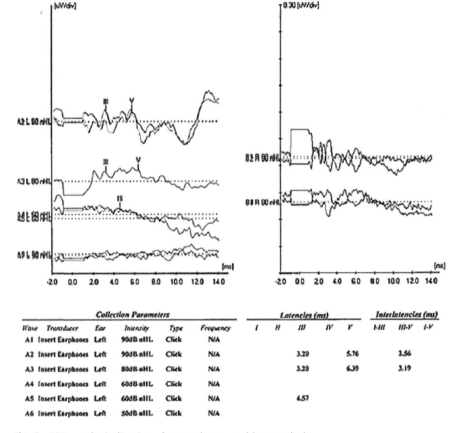

Fig. 5. ABR results indicating abnormal retrocochlear pathology

Click stimulus Left ear: rarefaction and condensation polarities were used at 80 dB nHL and a wave III and V were measured. Response at 60 dB nHL revealed a measurement of wave III (cochlear nucleus) but no recordable measurement of wave V (lateral lemniscus).

Auditory brainstem response test results/recommendations

Auditory brainstem response (ABR) results indicate electrophysiologic evidence of normal or near-normal cochlear function and absent or abnormal auditory pathway transduction. DPOAEs were present for both ears. The results indicate retrocochlear hearing loss, bilaterally. ABR is a test of cochlear/auditory nerve function and is not a test of hearing. Behavioral audiometric testing should be attempted to fully assess the entire auditory system including cognition of sound, and to support today's findings.

Ear, nose, and throat evaluation and recommendations

Physical examination was within normal limits. Recommendation was for an MRI and hearing aid trial. If no benefit was obtained from the hearing aids, cochlear implantation will be considered.

MRI completed (19 months)
MRI results indicated that baby boy had a stroke in utero, which likely caused retro-cochlear pathology.

Patient safety risk issue

- Failure to evaluate entire auditory system resulted in delay in treatment/communication abilities.

EXAMPLE 2: CHRONIC MIDDLE EAR DYSFUNCTION PATIENT
Clinical History

Patient X was seen for initial evaluation at 2 years of age after failed newborn hearing screening. Delayed follow-up is due to life-threatening issues taking precedence. Patient X has a medical history complicated by prematurity (born at 34 weeks) with extended neonatal ICU stay and genetics findings significant for chromosome 2q.37 deletion syndrome. Additional diagnosis significant for hypertension, reactive airway disease, subglottic stenosis, hydrocephalus, gastric tube feeds, global developmental delays, autism, Chiari I malformation, and visual deficits.

Audiological Testing

Initial results: no reliable pure tone results obtained, due to difficulty conditioning to complete the task; however, speech awareness threshold was found at 40-dB hearing level (**Fig. 6**). Middle ear status was significant for bilateral middle ear dysfunction or occlusion of external auditory canal.

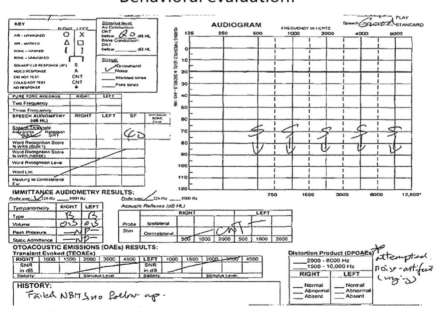

Fig. 6. Audiogram indicating bilateral middle ear dysfunction.

Patient X was referred for diagnostic ABR under general anesthesia (**Fig. 7**).
Patient received medical clearance and was fit for hearing aids fit based on ABR results. No middle ear assessment or bone conduction was completed prior to fitting.

```
EVOKED RESPONSE CONSULTATION REPORT:
BRAINSTEM AUDITORY EVOKED RESPONSE RESULTS:

LEFT CLICK THRESHOLD:  V wave was elicited up to 50 dB.
LEFT 4 KHZ TONE THRESHOLD:  V wave was elicited up to 60 dB.
LEFT 1 KHZ TONE THRESHOLD:  V wave was elicited up to 50 dB.
LEFT 500 HZ TONE THRESHOLD:  V wave was elicited up to 70 dB.
LEFT BONE CONDUCTION:  Not done


RIGHT CLICK THRESHOLD:  V wave was elicited at 60 dB.
RIGHT 4 KHZ TONE THRESHOLD:  V wave was elicited at 60 dB.
RIGHT 1 KHZ TONE THRESHOLD:  V wave was elicited up to 60 dB.
RIGHT 500 HZ TONE THRESHOLD:  V wave was elicited up to 70 dB.
RIGHT BONE CONDUCTION:  Not done


IMPRESSION:  This is an abnormal brainstem auditory evoked response indicative of bilateral hearing
loss.  Bone conduction was not performed.  ENT and Audiology evaluation is recommended.
```

Fig. 7. ABR results depicting moderate hearing loss.

Audiological testing continued to show middle ear dysfunction for the next 2 years with no intervention. At age 6 years old, testing suggested hearing loss to be conductive in nature. Pressure equalization tube placed at age 7 years and repeat ABR testing was completed after tube placement (**Fig. 8**).

ABR results at that time were consistent with normal hearing 500 Hz to 4000 Hz, bilaterally. Hearing aid use was ceased at that time.

Behavioral testing at 6 y of age:

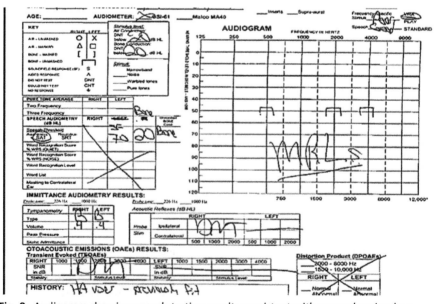

Fig. 8. Audiogram showing speech testing results consistent with severe hearing loss.

Patient Safety Concerns

- Full battery not used
- Hearing aids fit based on incomplete results
- Empower parents
- Use team approach to patient care
- Consider bone conduction hearing aids to avoid risk of over-amplification
- Frequent monitoring with durable medical equipment devices

EXAMPLE 3: MEDICALLY COMPLEX PATIENT
Clinical History

Patient Y has a birth history significant for born at 24 weeks, extremely low birth weight, microcephaly, severe spastic quadriparetic cerebral palsy, and complex partial epilepsy. Medical history is significant for acute respiratory failure, chronic lung disease of prematurity, complex partial epilepsy, delayed puberty, gastrostomy, generalized intestinal dysmotility, neuromuscular scoliosis, osteopenia, encephalopathy, pneumatosis intestinalis, respiratory failure, spastic cerebral palsy, tracheostomy tube, cortical visual impairment, and chronic middle ear dysfunction.

Audiological Testing

Patient Y has lived a state institution his entire life. At 2 years, results suggested no worse than a moderate hearing loss, for at least 2000 Hz, for at least the better hearing ear, if an ear difference should exist. No worse than a severe hearing loss, for at least some of the speech frequencies, in at least the better hearing ear, if an ear difference should exist. Pure tone and speech testing were evaluated but OAEs were not completed at that time. Tympanometry indicated normal middle ear function, and acoustic reflexes could not be tested due to patient movement (**Fig. 9**).

ABR was completed while the patient was under general anesthesia for pressure equalization tube placement with an ear, nose, and throat (ENT) physician. Standard setting was used. Results found no response to the limit of the equipment for click stimulus through air and bone conduction, consistent with severe to profound sensorineural hearing loss, bilaterally.

This patient was fit with hearing aid amplification prescribed to levels of ABR testing results. Several issues can be found with this logic.

1. Patient suffers from severe neurologic involvement, which may compromise ability of auditory system to respond to standard stimulus. ABR is likely not the best test to evaluate this patient's auditory system.
2. Failure to evaluate inner ear (OAEs) when middle ear system was clear.
3. Discounting behavioral results. In short, cross-check principle was not used.

Follow-up hearing evaluation at 10 years of age revealed that minimum response levels for unaided testing found pure tone testing results at severe to moderately severe hearing loss level. Speech response found at moderately severe hearing loss

Observation during behavioral evaluation:

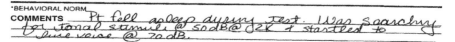

Fig. 9. Comments section on behavioral testing results.

level. OAEs were absent for the range of hearing where amplification was provided and were present starting at the frequencies that amplification rolls off (**Fig. 10**).

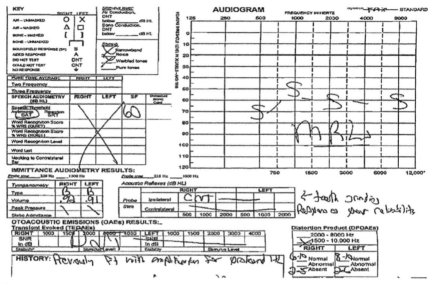

Fig. 10. Behavioral evaluation.

Patient Safety Concerns

- Full battery not used—failure to use cross-check principle.
- Patient's reaction to hearing aids was ignored by nurses, caregivers, and audiologist.
- If a patient continues to reject hearing aid amplification, the audiologist should always inquire further to ensure proper fit.

EXAMPLE 4 BACTERIAL MENINGITIS PATIENT
Clinical History

Patient X is 10 years old, a previously healthy girl who was admitted to the hospital for pneumococcal meningitis in the setting of acute sinusitis, which progressed to cerebritis and left-sided weakness, including left facial droop as well as left upper and lower extremity weakness.

The patient was seen by otolaryngology on hospital day 6 after some clinical worsening on broad-spectrum intravenous antibiotics. Given the concerning clinical picture and significant sinus disease (left side worse than right), the patient was taken to the operating room for image-guided endoscopic left ethmoidectomy and left frontal sinusotomy for persistent disease in these sinuses. At time of examination by ENT, patient was noted to have right beating nystagmus as well as left cranial nerve (CN) VII weakness (House-Brackmann score 2/6). She did not have any subjective hearing complaints at this time. At time of discharge, patient's hearing was intact subjectively to tuning fork bilaterally. CN VII had recovered by then too, and the only remaining cranial nerve deficit was sustained nystagmus with right extraocular movement. She also had continued, although somewhat improved, left upper and lower extremity weakness.

The patient was then discharged to inpatient rehabilitation program and later to home. Patient followed-up with pediatrician and, at that time, reported inability to hear out of the left ear since the time of discharge from the hospital as well as sustained nonpulsatile tinnitus on this side.

Audiological testing was done 23 days after discharge from the hospital.

AUDIOLOGICAL TESTING

Normal hearing for the right ear. Profound sensorineural hearing loss for the left ear.

Behavioral testing was completed using conventional methodology. DPOAEs and acoustic reflexes were consistent with behavioral results. Tympanometry revealed normal middle ear function, bilaterally.

Patient Safety Concerns

- Among patients with bacterial meningitis, 5% to 35% develop permanent sensorineural hearing loss, which is profound and bilateral in up to 4% of patients.[6] Audiological testing is imperative in all patients diagnosed with this disease, as soon as medically stable.
- Develop a national and international protocol to initiate hearing evaluation after bacterial meningitis, preferably before discharge from the hospital in all survivors of meningitis.

SUMMARY

Audiologists work with a team of talented and knowledgeable professionals in health care settings, including otolaryngologists, speech-language pathologists, and nurses. The role of audiologists in facilitating and strengthening a culture of patient safety is critical for hospitals. Patient safety includes individual, systemic, and institutional parameters. It is important for audiologists to clearly understand their role with the patient, the patient's data, and the policies and procedures in the hospital. The integration of these elements in a formal systematic approach for all hospital staff is critical to developing and sustaining a culture of patient safety within the hospital. Using the quality-improvement system to inform where changes are necessary and effective is important.

REFERENCES

1. American Speech-Language-Hearing Association. 2016 Audiology survey. Survey summary report: Number and type of responses. 2016. Available at: https://www.asha.org/uploadedFiles/2016-Audiology-Survey-Number-and-Type-of-Responses.pdf. Accessed September 12, 2018.
2. Saccone P, Steiger J. Audiologists' professional satisfaction. Am J Audiol 2012;21: 140–8.
3. Kirpalani S, LeFevre F, Phillips C, et al. Deficits in communication and information transfer between hospital-based and primary care physicians: implication for patient safety and continuity of care. JAMA 2007;297(8):831–41.
4. Jerger JF, Hayes D. The cross check principle in pediatric audiometry. Arch Otolaryngol 1976;102(10):614–20.
5. Hall J III. Crosscheck principle in pediatric audiology today: a 40-year perspective. J Audiol Otol 2016;20(2):59–67.
6. Merkus P, Free RH, Mylanus EA, et al. Dutch Cochlear Implant Group (CI-ON) consensus protocol on postmeningitis hearing evaluation and treatment. Otol Neurotol 2010;31(8):1281–6.

Patient Safety and Quality for Office-Based Procedures in Otolaryngology

Prerak D. Shah, MD

KEYWORDS

- Patient safety • Risk assessment • Office-based procedures • Complications
- Managing emergencies • Ambulatory

KEY POINTS

- Before performing an office-based procedure, judicious evaluation of patient and procedure risk factors should be completed, and a detailed procedure-specific informed consent should be obtained.
- Measures to prepare for emergencies include team role assignments and routine simulations, crash cart maintenance, and medication inventory.
- Most common and impactful procedure-related complications can include wrong site/side of surgery, airway obstruction, bleeding, and vasovagal syncope.
- Postprocedure monitoring of recovery should be routine and commensurate to invasiveness and risk associated with each specific procedure and patient.
- Sterilization of instruments, specimen handling, and medical documentation are postprocedure issues that need established, standardized protocols for all providers and office staff members.

INTRODUCTION

The shared mission to achieve greater value in health care is transforming the modern medical landscape and consequently changing the practice pattern of Otolaryngologists. This transformation has primarily been driven by efforts geared toward lowering the cost of health care and, to a lesser extent, an impetus of improving the quality of the delivered care. As a procedure-oriented specialty, Otolaryngologists have a unique opportunity to further enhance the value-based care offered in this new era of cost-containment, shared risk, and care coordination. There has been a substantial shift from procedure performance in hospitals and ambulatory surgery centers (ASCs)

Disclosure Statement: The author has no financial relationship with any commercial entity or any conflict of interest with the subject matter presented in this article.
New England Ear, Nose and Throat Center & Facial Plastic Surgery, Harvard Medical School, Massachusetts Eye and Ear Infirmary, 198 Massachusetts Avenue, Suite 103, North Andover, MA 01845, USA

Otolaryngol Clin N Am 52 (2019) 89–102
https://doi.org/10.1016/j.otc.2018.08.015   oto.theclinics.com

to office-based practices for several reasons, some of which include (1) regulatory and systematic inefficiencies of in-hospital procedures, (2) innovations in medical technology and surgical instrumentation, and (3) demand for greater cost and time efficiency by providers, patients, and payers[1] (**Box 1**).

In 2009, more than 12 million office-based procedures were performed in the United States, reflecting a precipitous increase in volume with a forecasted trajectory of continued growth.[2] The substantial shift to office-based procedures has outpaced the ability of local, state, and federal regulatory agencies to track outcomes and complications to the same extent that hospitals and ASCs are monitored.[2,3] Regulatory agencies facilitate the use of quality assurance methodologies and patient safety measures to improve quality of care and reduce negative outcomes.[4] In Florida, there was a 12.8 times greater risk of adverse incidents and death from office-based procedures compared with ASC patients with a mortality of 9.2 deaths per 100,000 patients with office-based procedures.[5] A recent claims-based study found that almost half of the office-based procedural complications were preventable if improvements were made in patient monitoring.[6] Office-based procedures present a higher-risk setting with reduced access to surgical equipment, emergency supplies and medication, less availability of trained ancillary staff, presence of office-related distractions, and, oftentimes, simultaneous patient visits during procedures. Procedures performed in an Otolaryngology office present an even greater risk as they involve manipulation of the airway and also have the potential for significant bleeding-related complications due to the abundant vascularity of the head and neck. Developing office-based patient safety strategies and best practice standards using evidence-based methods is essential as the specialty enters the domain of high-quality, value-based health care.[7]

The primary focus of this article is on patient safety and quality as they relate to office-based procedures in Otolaryngology. Most of these procedures are performed with the use of topical and/or local anesthesia alone, although there is an increasing trend toward performing more invasive office-based surgeries with concomitant use of anxiolytics, intravenous sedation, or even general anesthesia. Discussions regarding the safety and quality practices of office-based procedures using sedation or general anesthesia are certainly pertinent and of great importance but are outside the scope of this article. The remainder of the article is divided to match the normal sequence of in-office procedures, including preprocedural planning, procedural execution, and postprocedural follow-up.

Box 1
Contributing factors that have shifted procedures to an office-based setting

- Less facility and overhead costs compared with hospitals and ASCs
- Improved physician reimbursement
- Time-efficiency for patients and physicians
- Ease of scheduling and improved flexibility for patients and physicians
- Control of capital costs and equipment utilization by physicians

Data from Urman RD, Shapiro FE. Improving patient safety in the office: the Institute for Safety in Office-Based Surgery. In: The Anesthesia Patient Safety Foundation Newsletter. 2011. Available at: https://www.apsf.org/newsletters/html/2011/spring/02_officesafety.htm. Accessed March 17, 2018; and Mandel LM. Incorporating office-based otolaryngology procedures into your practice. In: Ear Nose Throat J. 2017. Available at: https://www.entjournal.com/whitepaper/incorporating-office-based-otolaryngology-procedures-your-practice. Accessed March 18, 2018.

PREPROCEDURAL PLANNING
Patient and Procedure Selection

The most critical decision in this process is the judicious selection of which patients and what procedures are safe and appropriate to be done in an office setting. An oversight or error in this process can result in unintended complications and patient harm. The current health care environment has incentivized performing higher-risk procedures on higher risks patients in office-based settings without many protective regulations on patient safety and quality.[5] Patient selection starts with a thorough preprocedure history and physical examination with a special focus on identifying risk factors that may potentially impact the safety and success of an in-office procedure. The timing of this evaluation is important because it should be completed early enough to obtain clearance from primary care providers or other medical specialists, optimize medical comorbidities, review supporting documentation, and obtain any necessary testing that may help lower the risk profile of the patient. Otolaryngologists should be vigilant of those patients who have not been regularly followed by their primary care providers because they may have undiagnosed or undermanaged comorbidities, such as hypertension or diabetes.[4] Medical risk factors should be screened for during the clinical evaluation, including any history of cardiac or pulmonary disease, bleeding problems, underlying obstructive sleep apnea, drug allergies, and procedure-related anxiety. The preprocedure examination should identify any challenging anatomic features, such as an assessment of the patient's airway and body mass index, which may preclude the ability to perform the procedure in an office setting.[3,4] Most hospitals and ASCs use the American Society of Anesthesiologists (ASA) Physical Status Classification System to risk-stratify patients for surgery, which can also be effective for in-office procedures (**Table 1**).[8] Patients who are ASA class I and II are deemed appropriate for in-office treatment, and provider discretion is used for higher ASA class patients based on the invasiveness and overall risk of the planned procedure.[9] For example, many Otolaryngology procedures that are minimally or mildly invasive with a low risk of complications can be done safely and appropriately in an ASA class III patient with judicious planning and preparation. **Table 2** includes a list of common Otolaryngology procedures stratified by risk and invasiveness of the procedure per the author's judgment. (No peer-reviewed classification of such risks exists for ambulatory practices.) Patients who are ASA class 3 and ASA class 4 who are planning a moderate-risk to high-risk office-based procedure may benefit from a more controlled setting in a hospital or ASC with more accessible Anesthesia personnel, improved ancillary support staff, and improved monitoring capabilities.

Table 1	
American Society of Anesthesiologists physical status classification system	
ASA Class	**Definition**
ASA I	Normal healthy patient
ASA II	A patient with mild systemic disease (smoker, well-controlled diabetes)
ASA III	A patient with severe systemic disease (poorly controlled diabetes, chronic obstructive pulmonary disease)
ASA IV	A patient with severe systemic disease that is a constant threat to life (recent [<3 mo] stroke or heart attack)
ASA V	A moribund patient who is not expected to survive without the operation
ASA VI	A declared brain dead patient

Table 2
Common office-based otolaryngology procedures stratified by extent of invasiveness and risk of complications

Invasiveness/Risk Level	Procedure
Low	Cerumen removal
	Division of tongue tie
	Flexible laryngoscopy
	Fine needle aspiration biopsy
	Intranasal biopsy
	Mastoid debridement
	Nasal endoscopy
	Nasopharyngoscopy
	Oral cavity biopsy
	Punch biopsy
	Removal of foreign body from ear
	Skin biopsy
	Tracheobronchoscopy (via tracheostomy tube)
Low to moderate	Botox and filler injection
	Control of epistaxis and nasal cautery
	Myringotomy ± tympanostomy tube
	Nasal polypectomy
	Oropharynx biopsy
	Removal of foreign body from nose
	Sialoendoscopy/sialolithotomy
	Transtympanic steroid injection
	Videostroboscopy
Moderate	Balloon-assisted sinus dilation
	Endoscopic nasopharynx biopsy
	Incision & drainage (I&D) auricular hematoma
	I&D facial abscess or superficial neck abscess
	I&D peritonsillar abscess
	Inferior turbinate reduction/cautery
	Postoperative sinus debridement
Moderate to high	Flexible laryngoscopy with biopsy
	Flexible laryngoscopy with injection
	Functional endoscopic sinus surgery

The complicated matrix of decision making based on the invasiveness and risks of the procedure and the myriad of patient-specific factors is ultimately what determines the appropriateness of choosing an office-based approach and, in the end, rests on the Otolaryngologist.

Consent

The process of procuring an informed consent before any procedure is fully engrained in the culture of hospitals and ASCs and widely accepted by surgeons; however, it remains largely unknown to what extent this is practiced in the office setting, particularly with regard to thoroughness and consistency. According to the Physician Insurers of American Association, approximately 6% of claims are brought forward due to lack of consent, which makes this not just an ethical obligation but also a legal duty.[10] Informed consent is the acknowledgment of the dialogue between a physician and patient reviewing the various aspects of the proposed procedure, including the indications, expectations, risks, and benefits of the procedure and the alternative options.

Several studies showed that 18% to 45% of surgical patients were unable to recall major risks of a planned surgery after signing consent, underscoring the potential limits of health literacy in surgical patients.[11] The language in this dialogue should be composed of nonmedical terminology, written and spoken at a fifth-grade level and interpreted/translated into the patient's primary language of communication.[10,11] Assessing patients' understanding of the planned procedure before signing the document is accomplished by having them repeat what was discussed in their own words, which can then be corrected or further discussed if warranted.[11]

The variety and volume of different procedures performed in an Otolaryngologist's office present challenges to the conventional process of obtaining informed consent. Many practices have patients sign a general "consent-to-treat" form at the time of registration for their appointment. For low-risk, minimally invasive procedures, many Otolaryngologists continue to have the physician-patient dialogue regarding the planned procedure and obtain verbal consent to the procedure, but not necessarily a signed procedure-specific informed consent document like in hospitals or ASCs. Vermal consent may be an acceptable practice for low-risk procedures listed in **Table 2** as long as the pertinent details are discussed with the patient and the specifics of the dialogue are included in the documentation of the procedure. More invasive procedures and those associated with greater risk of complications should ideally be performed in the conventional manner with a procedure-specific informed consent form signed by the patient and physician. Obtaining a signed informed consent will not eliminate the chance of a malpractice claim, but it is hoped that having had a detailed and comprehensive discussion and dialogue with the patient will minimize the likelihood.[10]

Procedure Team

A coordinated and integrated team approach is a prerequisite for improving outcomes and minimizing complications in any medical procedural intervention, which holds true in the office setting as well. Although most office-based procedures performed by Otolaryngologists usually occur in an examination or procedure room without any ancillary staff present, identifying team members and assigning their respective duties are critical to establishing consistency and efficiency. Staff educators should be familiarized with their role and function far in advance of the procedure. They oftentimes will help reaffirm any details of the procedure with the patient, answer any further questions, and offer guidance with reassurance. Staff members assigned the duties of greeting and preparing patients can be a tremendous source of encouragement by dispelling any preprocedure anxiety and stress.[9] For procedures using multiple devices, such as balloon-assisted sinus dilation, having a first assist may alleviate some of the hand-occupying and time-occupying burdens placed on the surgeon. In the event of an emergency, staff members should be aware of who makes the call for Emergency Medical Services (EMS), who stays nearby the physician and patient, who retrieves any necessary emergency equipment and supplies, and who will act as the point of contact to family members and other individuals affected by this. A staff member can also be assigned to monitor the patient during the recovery phase if indicated and to contact them later in the day after completion of the procedure to check on their status.

Code Cart

Although proper safety and resuscitative equipment is mandated in hospital and ASC settings, there are no requirements to have them accessible in a medical office setting.[4] From an Otolaryngologist's perspective, with the multitude of office-based procedures that are typically performed, having access to a fully equipped and maintained crash cart may prove to be an invaluable investment. Many medical offices are inadequately prepared to manage in-office emergencies. The most common reasons cited for this lack of preparedness are due to the infrequency of these events, time and financial constraints, and the close proximity of a local hospital to the office.[12] In the untoward event of an airway or cardiac emergency during a procedure, waiting for EMS to transport the patient to a local hospital may result in an untimely delay in instituting resuscitative efforts. **Box 2** includes some of the common components of an office-based crash cart.[4,12] A crash cart should be portable and stored in an accessible location because patient emergency locations can be variable.[12] Inventory of supplies and medications for used, missing or expired items, and maintenance of equipment should routinely be done to avoid untimely complications during a true emergency.[4]

Emergency Simulation

Just as important as having the necessary equipment and team members, scheduling routine simulations of emergency events can be one way to ensure optimal coordination of actions and maintenance of supply. The office staff should be familiar with the location of all emergency equipment and set up scheduled inventory of the crash cart equipment and medications.[4] A written protocol listing a stepwise approach to handling office emergencies and ideal arrival points for EMS will serve as a useful reference to office staff. Assigning specific duties to the appropriate staff members is a critical measure that should be reinforced on a routine basis (**Box 3**).

PROCEDURAL EXECUTION
Sterile Technique

Hospital and ASC settings have established protocols for infection control, sterility, and patient preparation before surgical intervention to minimize risks of nosocomial and postoperative infections. The expansive range of office-based procedures within Otolaryngology creates a wide potential for infection risk, therefore necessitating the appropriate level of aseptic technique for each procedure by the provider.[13] When hands are visibly soiled, soap and water should be used initially, and then the preferred method of hand hygiene according to the Centers for Disease Control and Prevention (CDC) and the World Health Organization is with use of an alcohol-based hand sanitizer.[14] Alcohol-based hand sanitizers have a broad-spectrum antimicrobial profile, improved compliance, better accessibility, and less irritation to the hands.[13,14] For procedures with clean wounds, such as an excisional skin biopsy of the face, antiseptic skin preparation is performed before the procedure, and proper aseptic technique with sterile gloves, sterile field, and sterile instrumentation should be used.[13] For clean-contaminated wounds, a clean technique with appropriate hand hygiene and use of clean gloves is recommended for a procedure such as biopsy of a lesion in the oropharynx. Universal precautions and use of personal protective equipment should be followed especially in cases where there is contact with blood or body fluid, mucous membranes, nonintact skin, or potentially infectious material.[14]

Anesthesia (Topical/Local)

One of the most important determinants of success with office-based procedures is minimizing and controlling the patient's level of pain. The advances in the delivery and safety of topical and local anesthetics have greatly improved the ability to perform invasive procedures in an office setting. Cocaine is one of the oldest topical anesthetics used in Otolaryngology, which has the beneficial effect of numbing exposed

---

Box 2
Components of emergency crash cart in the ambulatory setting

Equipment

Bag mask ventilator

Blood pressure cuff (multiple sizes)

Glucose meter

Intraosseous needle (18 g and 16 g)

Intravenous cather/butterfly needles (24 g to 18 g)

Intravenous extension tubing and T-connectors

Nasal airway (trumpet)

Nasogastric tubes

Non-rebreather

Oxygen mask

Oxygen tank and flow meter

Packing material: gauze

Portable suction device and catheters/Yankauer

Pulse oximetry

Stethoscope

Surgical airway set with endotracheal tubes

Universal precautions (gloves, masks, eye protection)

Medications

Aspirin

Decadron

Dextrose 25%

Diphenhydramine (oral and parental)

Epinephrine (1:1,000, 1:10,000)

Flumazenil

Naloxone (Narcan)

Nitroglycerine spray

Normal saline

Data from Appold K. Preparing for adverse events when performing office-based procedures. In: ENT Today. 2015. Available at: http://www.enttoday.org/article/preparing-for-adverse-events-when-performing-office-based-procedures/. Accessed March 17, 2018; and Toback SL. Medical emergency preparedness in office practice. Am Fam Physician 2007;75(11):1679–84.

---

tissue and acts as a potent vasoconstrictor to minimize bleeding from the tissue. Prior reports of adverse effects, primarily cardiac in nature, and the challenges of cost and safe storage have driven many Otolaryngologists to use alternative options, such as oxymetazoline with lidocaine, specifically in patients with heart disease.[15] Absorption of topical anesthesia is greatest in the face and scalp region and oftentimes can achieve a similar analgesic effect as injectable local anesthesia.[16] A known example of topical anesthesia without use of injectable local anesthesia is with phenol

---

Box 3
Assigned roles during acute office emergency

- Identify lead physician to respond to patient emergency
- Assist physician with patient care needs
- Bring crash cart when needed to patient
- Contact and direct EMS upon arrival
- Obtain initial set of vital signs
- If oxygen saturation is less than 93%, start oxygen by face mask
- Prepare and dispense any required medications
- Solicit other physicians and/or providers for assistance
- Inform waiting patients of possible delays
- Comfort and update any family members if present
- Contact family if not present

Data from Toback SL. Medical emergency preparedness in office practice. Am Fam Physician 2007;75(11):1679–84.

---

application on the tympanic membrane for minor ear drum procedures.[17] Many office-based laryngology and esophagology procedures are also routinely performed with only topical agents providing adequate anesthesia to suppress the patient's gag reflex, coughing, and risk of laryngospasm.

Most Otolaryngology procedures will use injectable local anesthetics to minimize any patient discomfort and can often be given following application of a topical anesthetic to lessen the needle-related pain. The wide variety of local anesthetics agents available allows for options for use based on specific needs such of the procedure and patient, such as onset and duration of action, toxicity, and effectiveness. Lidocaine with or without epinephrine is the most commonly used agent with recommendations of maximum doses of 7 mg/kg of lidocaine (if with epinephrine) and 4.5 mg/kg of lidocaine (if without epinephrine) for adults,[16] and for children, doses of 3 to 4.5 mg/kg of lidocaine (if with epinephrine) and 1.5 mg to 2 mg/kg of lidocaine (if without epinephrine). The use of bupivacaine and tetracaine helps provide longer duration of analgesia up to twice as long as lidocaine.[16] The vasoconstrictive action of epinephrine, usually used in concentrations of 1:100,000 and 1:200,000, helps reduce any bleeding but also decreases the mobilization of the anesthetic, thus increasing its duration of action and the dose tolerance of lidocaine. The concern for using epinephrine in areas such as the ears and nose leading to tissue necrosis has not been substantiated in multiple systematic reviews and randomized controlled trials.[16,18] Buffering the local anesthetic with the addition of sodium bicarbonate in order to increase the pH significantly reduces the pain during infiltration by about 20% to 40%.[16]

Inventory and Equipment

Maintaining equipment and checking inventory of medications used for office-based procedures should be routinely performed by the office staff or provider. Creating a checklist of task items is a simple, reliable, and effective means of ensuring the office is equipped for every patient before their procedure date. Some of the items of the checklist include the following:

- Checking expiration dates for all medications provided in the office
- Ensure adequate supply if additional medication required during the procedure
- Evaluate for contamination or damage to any bottles/containers
- Assess inventory of medication specifically for any controlled substances
- Follow manufacturer's recommendations on maintenance on all equipment
- Assess inventory and supply of disposable items required for procedures
- Recheck emergency crash cart

Complications

Complications are an inevitable risk of any procedure or surgery. The ultimate objective is to eliminate preventable complications and reduce the negative outcomes of unavoidable complications. The office setting creates a potentially challenging venue for managing unexpected complications, and taking measures to minimize these occurrences should be prioritized and instituted.

Wrong Site/Wrong Side

Wrong site and wrong side surgery have devastating consequences to both patient and providers and has resulted in many hospitals and ASCs in instituting mandatory marking of patient site and side of surgery in their respective preoperative areas. This marking is again reverified when performing the time-out before surgery in the operating room by the entire surgical team. With office-based procedures, similar standards should be maintained and followed. As mentioned, a verbal and, for higher-risk procedures, a signed written consent should be performed before any procedure in the office setting. The site and side should be clearly documented on the form. It is often useful to implement a time-out before performing a procedure in the office, such as for in-office sinus procedures or an injection laryngoplasty, to ensure site and side of procedure are confirmed with the patient and staff and match the consent form as well as to increase situational awareness among the care delivery team.

Complications: Airway/Anaphylaxis

As airway specialists, Otolaryngologists have the expertise and skills to manage most airway complications; however, airway complications in an office setting can be potentially disastrous particularly when there has been inadequate preparation with insufficient equipment and a poorly trained staff. If airway procedures are being performed, such as with office-based laryngology or patients with head and neck cancer, the crash cart can be supplemented with different sized endotracheal tubes, tracheostomy tubes, oral/nasal airways, intubating laryngoscopes, and a cricothyroidotomy kit. If allergy evaluations and treatments are performed, setting up a treatment plan for a patient with a potential anaphylactic reaction should be delineated before initiating these services. The crash cart should be stocked with injectable epinephrine, intravenous fluids and needles, oxygen and mask/cannula, airway devices, and a blood pressure monitoring device (see **Box 2**).[19]

Complications: Bleeding

The robust supply of blood to the head and neck explains the greater risk of bleeding complications with many Otolaryngology procedures. Bleeding complications become even more problematic when they occur in difficult to access areas, such as the posterior nasal cavity, oropharynx, and larynx. Prevention and preparation are paramount in avoiding these potentially devastating complications. Prevention begins with identifying risk factors for bleeding by completing a thorough patient and family history and complete review of medications for aspirin, antiplatelet agents, nonsteroidal anti-inflammatory drugs, Warfarin, and other anticoagulants. Further workup, including laboratory studies or consultation with Hematology, can then be obtained before the procedure if necessary.[20] Preventive measures also include minimizing potential bleeding from tissue by use of either topical or injectable vasoconstrictors or both. Despite these preventative measures, bleeding can still be confronted and problematic; therefore, other hemostatic measures may be necessary. There are many options for hemostasis depending on the site of the bleeding and its accessibility. Some of these include chemical, electrical, or ultrasonic energy coagulation devices, absorbable and nonabsorbable packing material, and sutures and vascular clips for ligation. The specific management of bleeding complications during office-based procedures is beyond the scope of this article, but preemptive measures can be taken specifically in patients with significant bleeding risk factors.

Complications: Vasovagal Syncope

Vasovagal presyncope and vasovagal syncope are some of the most common complications confronted by the Otolaryngologist during office-based procedures. This reflex-type of syncope is commonly triggered by emotional stress and is typically preceded by a prodrome of classic symptoms (sweating, pallor, cold clammy skin, nausea, dizziness).[21] The underlying cause is not fully understood but an emotional stress-related vagal overactivation and sympathetic withdrawal leads to a drop in heart rate in addition to vasodilation and pooling of blood in the lower limbs and splanchnic area. A resultant reduction in venous return to the heart lowers cardiac output, which in turn results in cerebral hypoperfusion and lightheadedness and eventual syncope.[21,22] Prevention of this cascade of events underscores the importance of making sure patients are adequately hydrated before any intervention. Identification of prodromal symptoms by the provider is critical so intervention can take place before loss of compensation, cerebral hypoperfusion, and resultant syncope.[21] Initial conservative treatment includes physical counter maneuvers (PCMs).[21,22] In a multicenter randomized controlled study, these PCMs were found to be a risk-free, effective, and low-cost treatment.[22] These simple measures have been recommended as first-line steps in treating patients with vasovagal presyncopal episodes.[21,22] The maneuvers include handgrip, arm tensing, and calf squeezing, which should be done immediately when prodromal symptoms are identified. A modified version of PCMs is described in **Fig. 1** with the patient in the supine position.[21,22] These maneuvers can be repeated until symptoms dissipate and eventually resolve.[22]

POSTPROCEDURAL FOLLOW-UP
Recovery

The process of postoperative monitoring after a surgery is streamlined and inherent in the culture of hospitals and ASCs but not necessarily in the office setting. Because most office-based procedures are performed without general anesthesia or sedation, the need for postprocedure monitoring is not as evident, but patients should be evaluated after completion of any procedure to ensure their safe departure from the office. After completion of the procedure, an assessment should be performed by the Otolaryngologist or staff member to ensure there is not any unseen complications from the procedures or new symptoms that may warrant further investigation, such as chest pain, shortness of breath, or lightheadedness. Patients oftentimes will be either unable to recognize the importance of new symptoms especially after an intervention or may be fearful and unwilling to share these with the physician. Patients, specifically the ones who have driven themselves to the office, should only be released from the office

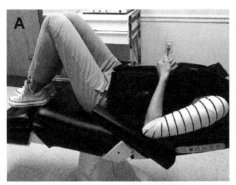
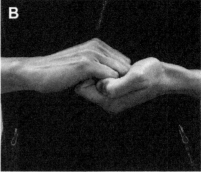
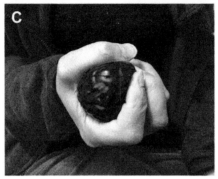

Fig. 1. (A–C) Modified physical counterpressure maneuvers. See Refs.[21,22] for further information. (A) Supine position and calf squeeze: -modified physical counterpressure maneuvers are initiated by placing the patient in a supine or Trendelenburg position to minimize risk of a fall. Bending the knee while squeezing the calf muscles and buttocks will help mobilize venous pooling in the lower extremities. (B) Arm tensing: gripping both hands and pulling away from each other tightly as shown can also be done simultaneously as another counterpressure maneuver. (C) Handgrip: An alternative option is to grasp a foam or rubber ball and squeeze it continuously until symptoms start to dissipate. (*Courtesy of* Julie Giordani, PA-C, North Andover, MA.)

once they have proven to be in a normal physical, cognitive, and mental state. If there is any concern for impairment, they should be kept in the procedure room with constant supervision by the physician or trained staff member until symptoms resolve or the emergency response algorithm has been initiated. Once a patient is stable and has been discharged, a follow-up communication later in the day can be a helpful and empathetic measure to answer any questions that may have come up since leaving the office.

Sterility and Instrument Sterilization

Recently there has been heightened interest within Otolaryngology regarding the appropriate method of disinfection, sterilization, and storage of in-office instruments intended for patient use.[14] In 2013, The Joint Commission identified 30% of office-based surgery sites noncompliant with their standards to reduce the risk of infection with medical equipment and instruments.[23] The potential transmission of disease from instrument contamination remains a primary concern with office-based procedures. Dedicated staff training and education of the established standards of sterilization and disinfection should be carefully performed. The 2008 CDC Guidelines for Disinfection and Sterilization for Healthcare Facilities have been adopted by many hospitals and ASCs and can be applied to the office setting as well.[24] Used instruments should be cleaned either manually or mechanically as soon as possible to remove any visible organic residue and soiling. From a sterility standpoint, there are 3 categories of disinfection by the CDC guidelines, including sterilization, high-level, and low-level disinfection.

- Sterilization: destroys all microbials and bacterial spores (surgical instruments) that enter normally sterile tissues or the vascular system
- High-level disinfection: instruments (endoscopes) that touch mucous membranes or nonintact skin
- Low-level disinfection: instruments (blood pressure cuffs/stethoscopes/environmental surfaces) that touch intact skin

A high-level disinfection as outlined by these guidelines should be performed for flexible and rigid endoscopes in the office, which have recently been implicated in noncompliance surveys.[24]

Specimen Handling

Tissue specimens and biopsies obtained in an operating room are sent to the pathology department in a very standardized fashion, where each step can be easily referenced and accounted for. This process should be simulated in the office setting with safeguards in place during each hand-off. Once a biopsy or excision is performed, the tissue specimen should be placed in a clearly labeled transport vial, which securely holds the appropriate fixative or storage medium. The vial label should include patient first and last name, date of birth, date of biopsy procedure, surgeon name, and site and side of biopsy at a minimum. Whether an office staff member or courier is transporting the specimen, the individuals who are responsible for handling of the specimen should readily be identified and be accountable for the specimen delivery. The consequences of a lost or mislabeled specimen can be longstanding with resultant patient dissatisfaction, patient harm, and even legal ramifications.[25] By simply implementing a standardized process for specimen handling along with clear communication and accountability with hand-offs, these mishaps can certainly be avoidable.

Documentation

The past decade has seen one of the most dramatic transformations in medical documentation ever seen in the health care arena. As most providers currently depend on electronic medical records, the use of templates for operative and procedure notes is commonplace and thus has necessitated a need to ensure all the pertinent details of a procedure are included in the documentation. Customarily, billing compliance does mandate adding sufficient details in a procedure note to justify the submitted billing code. The documentation should consistently include the indications and medical necessity, procedure-specific information (site, side, anesthesia, and technique), findings, specimens, complications, and patient tolerance. The greatest likelihood of recalling the specifics of the procedure is immediately after the procedure, which is the ideal time to document the details. Every patient and procedure will have differences worth noting; therefore, inclusion of all pertinent individualized points regarding the procedure is of utmost importance and could prove useful in the future from not only a continuity of care perspective but also a medicolegal one.

SUMMARY

Several proactive measures and preventative strategies can be implemented by Otolaryngologists to optimize patient outcomes and minimize the risk of procedure complications in the office setting. Developing a proficiency and comfort level with office-based procedures will become increasingly more important as the market forces are driving this shift within the rapidly changing world of health care. The systems that enhance patient safety and quality within hospital systems will need to be tailored to the office environment. One of the primary challenges and potential benefits in instituting these to office-based procedures is the lack of regulatory agencies that provide oversight and accreditation.[2] As the envelope continues to be pushed with higher-risk patients and more invasive procedures being performed in an office setting, the need to set standards for optimal quality care and for patient safety has never been greater.

REFERENCES

1. Urman RD, Shapiro FE. Improving patient safety in the office: The Institute for Safety in Office-Based Surgery. In: The Anesthesia Patient Safety Foundation Newsletter. 2011. Available at: https://www.apsf.org/newsletters/html/2011/spring/02_officesafety.htm. Accessed March 17, 2018.
2. Urman RD, Punwani N, Shapiro FE. Office-based surgical and medical procedures: educational gaps. Ochsner J 2012;12:383–8.
3. Stierer TL, Collop NA. Preoperative testing and risk assessment: perspectives on patient selection in ambulatory anesthetic procedures. Ambul Anesth 2015;2: 67–77.
4. Appold K. Preparing for adverse events when performing office-based procedures. In: ENT Today. 2015. Available at: http://www.enttoday.org/article/preparing-for-adverse-events-when-performing-office-based-procedures/. Accessed March 17, 2018.
5. Vila H, Soto R, Cantor AB, et al. Comparative outcomes analysis of procedures performed in physician offices and ambulatory surgery centers. Arch Surg 2003;138:991–5.
6. Domino KB. Office-based Anesthesia: lessons learned from the closed claims project. ASA Newsl 2001;65(6):9–11, 15.
7. Contrera KJ, Ishii LE, Setzen G, et al. Accountable care organizations and Otolaryngology. Otolaryngol Head Neck Surg 2015;153(2):170–4.
8. The American Society of Anesthesiologists Physical Status Classification System. 2014. Available at: https://www.asahq.org/resources/clinical-information/asa-physical-status-classification-system#. Accessed March 21, 2018.
9. Mandel LM. Incorporating office-based otolaryngology procedures into your practice. In: Ear Nose Throat J. 2017. Available at: https://www.entjournal.com/whitepaper/incorporating-office-based-otolaryngology-procedures-your-practice. Accessed March 18, 2018.
10. Morton R. Informed consent: substance and signature. 2013. Available at: https://www.thedoctors.com/articles/informed-consent-substance-and-signature/. Accessed March 21, 2018.
11. Wu HW, Nishimi RY, Page-Lopez CM. Implementing a national voluntary consensus standard for informed consent: a user's guide for healthcare professionals. In: National Quality Forum. 2005. Available at: http://www.qualityforum.org/Publications/2005/09/Implementing_a_National_Voluntary_Consensus_Standard_for_Informed_Consent__A_User_s_Guide_for_Healthcare_Professionals.aspx. Accessed March 21, 2018.

12. Toback SL. Medical emergency preparedness in office practice. Am Fam Physician 2007;75(11):1679–84.
13. Hunt J. Aseptic technique and clean technique procedure. In: Southern Health NHS Foundation Trust. 2014. Available at: http://www.southernhealth.nhs.uk/_resources/assets/inline/full/0/29049.pdf. Accessed March 21, 2018.
14. Centers for Disease Control and Prevention (CDC) Guide to infection prevention in outpatient settings: minimum expectations for safe care. 2016. Available at: https://www.cdc.gov/infectioncontrol/pdf/outpatient/guide.pdf. Accessed March 21, 2018.
15. Dwyer C, Sowerby L, Rotenberg BW. Is cocaine a safe topical agent for use during endoscopic sinus surgery? Laryngoscope 2016;126:1721–3.
16. Kouba DJ, LoPiccolo MC, Alam M, et al. Guidelines for the use of local anesthesia in office-based dermatologic surgery. J Am Acad Dermatol 2016;74(6):1201–19.
17. Sing T. Use of phenol in anaesthetizing the eardrum. Internet J Otorhinolaryngol 2005. Available at: http://ispub.com/IJORL/4/2/6276. Accessed March 21, 2018.
18. Häfner HM, Röcken M, Breuninger H. Epinephrine-supplemented local anesthetics for ear and nose surgery: clinical use without complications in more than 10,000 surgical procedures. J Dtsch Dermatol Ges 2005;3(3):195–9.
19. Lieberman P, Nicklas RA, Oppenheimer J. The diagnosis and management of anaphylaxis practice parameter: 2010 update. J Allergy Clin Immunol 2010; 126(3):477–80.
20. Thiele T, Kaftan H, Hosemann W, et al. Hemostatic management of patients undergoing ear-nose-throat surgery. GMS Curr Top Otorhinolaryngol Head Neck Surg 2015;(14):Doc07. Available at: https://www.ncbi.nlm.nih.gov/pmc/articles/PMC4702056/pdf/CTO-14-07.pdf. Accessed March 21, 2018.
21. Kenny RA, McNichols T. The management of vasovagal syncope. An International Journal of Medicine 2016;767–73.
22. Van Dijk N, Quartieri F, Blanc JJ, et al. Effectiveness of physical counterpressure maneuvers in preventing vasovagal syncope: the physical counterpressure manoeuvres trial (PC-Trial). J Am Coll Cardiol 2006;48(8):1652–7.
23. Available at: https://www.jointcommission.org/issues/article.aspx?Article=OnSN6wB9zLJ4d9rcQg%2Fkk23LJ5axbSViQF2x1VoLaKc%3D. Accessed March 28, 2018.
24. Rutala WA, Weber DJ, HICPAC. Guidelines for disinfection and sterilization in healthcare facilities. 2008. Available at: https://www.cdc.gov/infectioncontrol/pdf/guidelines/disinfection-guidelines.pdfd. Accessed March 21, 2018.
25. Shirey C, Perrego K. Standardizing the handling of surgical specimens. AORN J 2015;102(5):516.

Device Safety

Vinay K. Rathi, MD[a,b,*], Stacey T. Gray, MD[a,b]

KEYWORDS

- Medical device • Otolaryngology • FDA • Premarket approval • 510(k)
- Postmarket studies

KEY POINTS

- The type and strength of premarket evidence required by the US Food and Drug Administration (FDA) for device clearance or approval predominantly depends on device risk classification (low-risk, moderate-risk, or high-risk).
- Moderate-risk devices (eg, vocal fold injectables and ossicular prostheses) are cleared for marketing via the 51(k) pathway and typically do not require premarket clinical evidence of safety.
- High-risk devices (eg, cochlear implants and dermal fillers) are approved for marketing via the premarket approval pathway and require premarket clinical evidence providing reasonable assurance of safety and effectiveness.
- The FDA conducts both passive (adverse event reporting) and active (manufacturer-required studies) postmarket surveillance to address important safety questions (eg, long-term outcomes or rare adverse events).
- The FDA is currently developing advanced methods of postmarket surveillance that leverage clinically based data sources, which may include the society-sponsored otolaryngology registry in the future.

INTRODUCTION

Medical devices are essential in the diagnosis and treatment of otolaryngologic disease. The US Food and Drug Administration (FDA) is tasked with assuring the safety and effectiveness of these devices. Otolaryngologists, in turn, are often responsible for helping patients to understand risks, benefits, and alternatives when deciding whether a device should be used in their medical care. To best counsel patients, otolaryngologists should be aware of the strengths and limitations of device regulation by the FDA. This article provides an overview of the FDA regulatory framework for medical

Disclosure Statement: The authors have no conflicts of interest to disclose.
[a] Department of Otolaryngology–Head and Neck Surgery, Massachusetts Eye and Ear Infirmary, 243 Charles Street, Boston, MA 02114, USA; [b] Department of Otolaryngology, Harvard Medical School, Boston, MA, USA
* Corresponding author. Department of Otolaryngology–Head and Neck Surgery, Massachusetts Eye and Ear Infirmary, 243 Charles Street, Boston, MA 02114.
E-mail address: vinay_rathi@meei.harvard.edu

devices, premarket safety standards for marketing devices, and postmarket methods of safety surveillance. Future directions for monitoring device safety are reviewed as well.

US FOOD AND DRUG ADMINISTRATION REGULATORY FRAMEWORK

The Medical Device Amendments of 1976 first established a 3-tiered risk classification system for the regulation of medical devices.[1] Under this statute, the FDA categorizes devices into 1 of 3 classes (class I—low risk, class II—moderate risk, and class III—high-risk) (**Table 1**) based on the level of control necessary to assure safety and effectiveness.[2] These controls include general controls, special controls, and premarket approval (PMA) or humanitarian device exemption (HDE)[3]:

- General controls—basic provisions, such as good manufacturing practices, lawful labeling, and manufacturer registration with the FDA
- Special controls—device-specific controls necessary to assure safety and effectiveness, such as performance standards or special labeling requirements
- PMA/HDE—regulatory pathways requiring premarket clinical evidence of safety and effectiveness (PMA) or probable benefit (HDE)

Low-Risk (Class I) Devices

Approximately two-thirds of all medical devices are classified as low-risk.[4] These devices, with few exceptions, are subject only to general controls and do not undergo premarket review by the FDA. Otolaryngologic examples include devices, such as tongue depressors and otoscopes.

Moderate-Risk (Class II) Devices

Approximately one-third of devices are classified as moderate-risk.[4] These devices are subject to both general controls and special controls. To market moderate-risk devices, manufacturers must obtain FDA clearance via the 510(k) process.[5] Otolaryngologic examples include devices, such as ossicular prostheses and vocal fold implants.

High-Risk (Class III) Devices

Few (1%–2%) devices are classified as high-risk.[4] High-risk devices are defined as those that (1) support or sustain life, (2) are of substantial importance in preventing illness, or (3) present potentially unreasonable risk to patients.[6] High-risk devices are predominantly approved via the PMA pathway, which is the most rigorous method of FDA premarket review. For high-risk devices intended to diagnose or treat rare (affecting <8000 US patients per year) diseases, manufacturers may seek marketing authorization through the less rigorous HDE pathway[7]; no otolaryngologic devices have been approved via the HDE pathway to date.[8] Examples of high-risk devices include cochlear implants and dermal fillers.

PREMARKET SAFETY STANDARDS

The type (ie, nonclinical or clinical) and strength of premarket evidence required by the FDA predominantly depends on device risk classification. By law, the FDA may only compel manufacturers to provide the minimum amount of information necessary to assure safety and effectiveness.[9] As a result, low-risk and moderate-risk devices are typically cleared without supporting clinical evidence,[4,10,11] and high-risk devices are often approved on the basis of limited clinical studies.[12–15] Although this approach is intended to facilitate patient access to innovative technologies and is more stringent

Table 1
US Food and Drug Administration regulatory framework for medical devices

Device Class	Risk	Examples	Proportion[a]	Regulatory Controls	Review Pathway	Review Standard
Class I	Low-risk	Tongue depressor Otoscope	67%	General controls	None[b]	None
Class II	Moderate-risk	Ossicular prosthesis Vocal fold injection	31%	General controls and special controls (device-specific)	510(k) process[c]	"Substantial equivalence" to predicate device[d]
Class III	High-risk	Cochlear implant Dermal filler	1%	General controls and PMA	PMA	Clinical evidence of safety and effectiveness
			<1%	General controls and HDE	HDE [e]	Clinical evidence of safety and "probable benefit"

[a] Source: Institute of Medicine. Medical devices and the public's health: the FDA 510(k) clearance process at 35 years. 2011.
[b] Exceptions include select class I devices subject to 510(k) review.
[c] Exceptions include select class II devices exempt from 510(k) review.
[d] Exceptions include class I and class II devices without predicates subject to de novo review.
[e] Reserved for select class III devices indicated for the diagnosis or treatment of uncommon illnesses.

Reproduced from Rathi VK, Gadkaree SK, Ross JS, et al. US Food and Drug Administration clearance of moderate-risk otolaryngologic devices via the 510(k) process, 1997-2016. Otolaryngol Head Neck Surg 2017;157(4):608–17; with permission. ©American Academy of Otolaryngology—Head and Neck Surgery Foundation.

than European policy,[16,17] the FDA nonetheless has come under scrutiny in recent years after a series of high-profile recalls of unsafe devices, such as metal-on-metal hip replacement prostheses, pelvic mesh implants, and implantable cardioverter-defibrillators.[18–20]

510(k) Process

The 510(k) process requires manufacturers to demonstrate that a new or modified device is "substantially equivalent" to a previously cleared "predicate device" with respect to intended use and technological characteristics.[5] The FDA generally grants clearance on the basis of nonclinical evidence, such as bench testing and technical specifications.[4,10] Clinical evidence of safety and effectiveness is rarely required to validate substantial equivalence; just one-quarter of recently cleared otolaryngologic devices were supported by premarket clinical testing, which largely comprise small, uncontrolled studies.[11]

The 510(k) pr6ocess has earned much criticism in the wake of recent public health crises related to faulty devices.[18,19] Debate over the 510(k) process has centered around 6 key issues[21]:

1. Split predicates—manufacturers were historically permitted to market entirely novel devices on the basis of substantial equivalence to a combination of features derived from predicates with different intended uses and technological characteristics. For instance, the FDA cleared the first sinus balloon device in 2005 as an amalgam of a lacrimal dilator, a circular cutting punch, and an antrum curette.[22]
2. High-risk device exemptions—until recently, the FDA has allowed manufacturers to market certain high-risk devices, such as mandibular reconstruction plates,[23] via the 510(k) process. These devices were initially granted temporary exemption from more rigorous premarket review as a transitional measure under the Medical Device Amendments of 1976.[24]
3. Unsafe predicates—manufacturers may obtain clearance on the basis of substantial equivalence to unsafe predicates, including permanently recalled devices.[10] Few otolaryngologic devices cleared via the 510(k) process have been subject to FDA recall and none has been recalled for life-threatening or serious health hazards to date.[11]
4. Dissimilar predicates—permissive regulation has enabled manufacturers to obtain clearance for unproved new devices based on substantial equivalence to predicates with different intended uses and technological characteristics.[18,24,25]
5. Predicate creep—iterative device modification and application of substantial equivalence can result in the clearance of unproved new devices that differ substantially from better characterized predicates. For example, a calcium hydroxylapatite–based vocal fold implant was recently cleared without specific supporting clinical evidence. Clearance was based on a lineage of predicate devices originating in 1985 with a bovine bone graft indicated for dental and oromaxillofacial reconstruction.[11] Modified versions of existing devices (eg, design alterations or labeling updates in intended use) account for approximately half of all 510(k) clearances.[11]
6. Lack of transparency—premarket scientific data supporting FDA clearance of new devices are rarely accessible to help inform decision making by patients and physicians. In a recent study, performance data were not publicly available within FDA clearance summaries for more than 80% of otolaryngologic devices.[11]

Although most devices recalled for life-threatening or serious health hazards are marketed with 510(k) clearance, patients and physicians may have few legal options, because the US Supreme Court has ruled that substantial equivalence is not a determination of safety and effectiveness and manufacturers are exempt from tort litigation over device defects.[26,27] Given weaknesses of the system and lack of recourse against manufacturers, the National Academy of Medicine recommended that the FDA replace the 510(k) process with an entirely new regulatory framework for moderate-risk devices in 2011,[4] a directive that the agency is now seriously considering.[28] In the interim, the FDA has taken several steps to strengthen the 510(k) process, such as banning split predicates, prohibiting review of high-risk devices,[24] and increasing the public availability of scientific data.[29]

Premarket Approval

The PMA pathway requires manufacturers to submit clinical evidence providing reasonable assurance of safety and effectiveness to market new high-risk devices.[6] Manufacturers generate initial safety data through in vitro (phase I) and feasibility (phase II) studies, which may offer important insights to guide premarket development (eg, design modifications) and clinical use (eg, anatomic restrictions) and inform the design of pivotal (phase III) studies.[30] FDA premarket review of high-risk devices primarily centers on pivotal study results.[31]

In contrast to the United States, the European Union requires manufacturers only to demonstrate that high-risk devices perform "as intended" and are likely safe.[17] Although this less stringent approach facilitates earlier patient access to new technologies, devices first approved in the European Union are more likely to be subject to postmarket safety alerts and recalls.[16] Furthermore, no high-risk otolaryngologic devices have been recalled for life-threatening or serious health hazards to date.[15] Nonetheless, recent work has highlighted several important limitations in the premarket clinical evidence supporting FDA approval of high-risk devices:

1. Strength of evidence—unlike prescription drugs, which are typically approved on the basis of 2 randomized double-blind controlled trials,[32] high-risk devices are most often approved on the basis of a single pivotal clinical study without blinding, comparators, or clinical endpoints.[12–15] In addition, pivotal study follow-up is often limited in duration, despite the fact that many high-risk devices are designed for long-term implantation. Among implantable high-risk otolaryngologic devices, the median pivotal study follow-up was approximately 26 weeks.[15]

2. External validity—compared with drug trials, pivotal studies of devices are small[33]; enrollment is generally less than 120 patients for high-risk otolaryngologic devices.[15] Moreover, important patient groups, including women, children, the elderly, and minorities, are under-represented in pivotal studies.[34] To address this issue, the FDA has recently implemented initiatives to diversify enrollment and better understand device performance in these patients.[35]

3. Device modifications—after initial approval, manufacturers must submit supplemental applications to implement labeling, design, and manufacturing changes that have an impact on device safety and effectiveness.[36] Clinical data are typically required only for supplemental applications expanding device indications for use (eg, to include new patient populations).[37,38] Devices may undergo substantial postmarket modification via supplemental applications[37,39]; high-risk otolaryngologic devices often undergo more than 20 such changes.[38] Although supplemental applications may facilitate rapid iterative improvement in device performance, these modifications may also result in new versions that differ from the models originally evaluated in pivotal studies or result in unintended clinical consequences.[38,40–42]

POSTMARKET SAFETY SURVEILLANCE

Given constraints of premarket evaluation, the FDA has adopted a total product life-cycle approach to medical device regulation.[43] This approach enables the FDA to address uncertainties about device risks and benefits that are present at the time of approval or arise in the context of real-world use. This includes questions about long-term safety, rare adverse events, or new indications.[43,44] The FDA presently conducts both passive (ie, adverse event reporting) and active (ie, required clinical studies) postmarket surveillance, although both mechanisms have important limitations. The agency is also developing new methods to identify problematic devices and characterize product performance using clinically based data sources, such as claims, registries, and electronic health records.[44]

Adverse Event Reporting

The FDA conducts passive postmarket surveillance by monitoring adverse event reports submitted by manufacturers, health care facilities, and providers. All manufacturers and health care facilities (eg, hospitals) are required to report all deaths and serious adverse events attributable to known or suspected device malfunction.[45] In addition, the FDA has partnered with several hundred clinical sites (known as the Medical Product Safety Network) to collect complementary safety data (eg, close calls) and perform targeted surveillance.[46,47] Although providers and patients are not mandated to report adverse device events, the FDA MedWatch program enables voluntary electronic reporting of adverse events.[48] Patients, providers, and other interested parties (eg, researchers) may access adverse event reports through a publicly available online FDA database.[49] Although such reports may prove valuable in identifying safety concerns,[50] the FDA and others have noted that the utility of passive postmarket surveillance may be limited by several important factors:

1. Reporting quality—adverse event reports are not standardized and may be submitted by individuals unfamiliar with of the details of clinical care. As a result, reports often include insufficient information to identify devices and characterize adverse events.[51] Prior work in the field of otolaryngology has demonstrated that variable report quality may preclude meaningful systematic analysis of adverse device events.[52,53]
2. Under-reporting—many adverse events are never reported as a result of poor end-user engagement; less than 10% of adverse event reports are submitted by patients or providers, who may fail to identify potentially problematic devices, fear legal repercussions, or lack the capability to integrate reporting into clinical operations.[44,51]
3. Delayed/biased reporting—manufacturers decide whether adverse events are due to device malfunctions and need not report complications deemed unrelated. This may lead manufacturers to attribute events to other factors (eg, procedural error), minimize the severity of negative outcomes, or significantly delay reporting.[51,54] Furthermore, reporting by patients and providers may be biased by extraneous factors (eg, media coverage).[44]
4. Lack of denominator—prior to initial implementation of unique device identifiers by the FDA in 2014, there was no way to ascertain the total number of devices in clinical use. Along with under-reporting, this limitation precludes calculation of product-specific adverse event rates and hinders the detection of safety concerns.[51]

Despite current limitations of passive postmarket surveillance, adverse event reporting via MedWatch allows patients and clinicians to provide the FDA with real-world insights into device safety without fear of retribution. Given that federal certification criteria now require electronic health records to capture unique device identifiers for implantable technologies,[44] many providers may soon be enabled to contribute to surveillance efforts in the course of clinical practice.

Postmarket Studies

The FDA conducts active postmarket surveillance by requiring device manufacturers to conduct additional studies after initial clearance or approval. Depending on device risk classification and the question to be addressed, the FDA may order 2 types of postmarket studies:

1. 522 Postmarket Surveillance Studies (522 Studies)—these studies are typically initiated in response to safety concerns arising in the context of real-world use and may be ordered for up to 3 years in duration for both moderate-risk and high-risk devices that meet any of the following 4 criteria[55]:
   a. Failure likely resulting in serious adverse health consequences
   b. Expected significant use in pediatric populations
   c. Intended for implantation in the body for over a year
   d. Intended to be a life-sustaining or life-supporting device
      The FDA has ordered approximately 400 522 Studies to date.[56] Nearly all have examined moderate-risk devices cleared via the 510(k) pathway, with more than three-quarters examining metal-on-metal hip implants or pelvic meshes. Only one 522 Study has been initiated to evaluate an otolaryngologic device, a tympanostomy tube cleared for placement in pediatric patients under sedation[11]; this ongoing study was ordered in 2016 to assess the rate and risk factors for conversion to general anesthesia and has thus far progressed inadequately according to the FDA.[23]
      The potential for 522 Studies to inform FDA regulation and clinical practice has often been limited by significant delays in completion, which may occur as a result of insufficient enrollment, manufacturer incentives to minimize safety concerns, and difficulties finalizing research protocols (eg, due to disagreements between the FDA and manufacturers)[56,57]; nonetheless, the FDA rarely imposes penalties when manufacturers fail to meet postmarket study commitments.[44] Furthermore, given that 522 studies cannot extend beyond 3 years' duration, important questions about the long-term outcomes of devices cleared via the 510(k) process may remain unanswered.[57]

2. Post-Approval Studies (PAS)—these studies may be ordered as a condition of initial or supplemental approval for high-risk devices regulated via the PMA and HDE pathways.[58] In contrast to 522 Studies, PAS are not subject to limitations in duration and are intended to complement premarket understanding of device safety and effectiveness. Approximately two-thirds of PAS require prospective clinical data collection.[56]

The FDA has ordered PAS for approximately three-quarters of all high-risk otolaryngologic devices.[15] The majority of these PAS examined long-term outcomes or device performance in patient subgroups under-represented in premarket studies (eg, ethnic minorities and women). PAS may additionally help confirm clinical benefit for new devices. For instance, the FDA approved a hypoglossal nerve stimulator for the treatment of obstructive sleep apnea based on a pivotal study using surrogate primary endpoints (apnea-hypopnea index and oxygen desaturation index) on the condition that the manufacturer conduct a PAS evaluating quality of life measures.[15,59,60] Although PAS may greatly inform understanding of device safety (eg, by prompting manufacturers to withdraw faulty devices from the market), the utility of these studies can be limited by small enrollment numbers, delays in completion, and lack of publicly available findings.[61] Furthermore, PAS may not serve as a cost-effective means to assure device safety, given an estimated expenditure of $2 million per study and $150 million per year.[62]

FUTURE DIRECTIONS

As noted by the FDA,[44] traditional methods of premarket and postmarket evaluation may be inadequate to fully understand the risks and benefits of medical devices. Moreover, devices may often be subject to limited postmarket study by manufacturers or independent investigators outside of FDA requirements.[63,64] With these limitations in mind, the FDA recently launched the National Evaluation System for Health Technology, a public-private collaborative aimed at applying advanced analytics to real-world clinical data sources (eg, registries, electronic health records, and claims) to generate insight into device performance across the total product life cycle.[44] As the FDA develops enhanced methods of device evaluation, otolaryngologists should understand the current strengths and limitations of regulation and contribute to surveillance efforts (eg, via adverse event reporting or clinical study) to best promote the safe and effective use of these technologies. Moving forward, otolaryngologists may soon be able to leverage a society-sponsored clinical data registry to better promote safe and effective use of devices as part of this initiative.[65]

REFERENCES

1. U.S. Congress. Medical device amendments of 1976. 1976. Available at: https://www.gpo.gov/fdsys/pkg/STATUTE-90/pdf/STATUTE-90-Pg539.pdf. Accessed April 1, 2018.

2. U.S. Food and Drug Administration. Classify your medical device. 2018. Available at: http://www.fda.gov/MedicalDevices/DeviceRegulationandGuidance/Overview/ClassifyYourDevice/. Accessed April 1, 2018.

3. U.S. Food and Drug Administration. Regulatory controls. 2018. Available at: https://www.fda.gov/MedicalDevices/DeviceRegulationandGuidance/Overview/GeneralandSpecialControls/default.htm#special. Accessed April 1, 2018.

4. Institute of Medicine. Medical devices and the public's health: the FDA 510(k) clearance process at 35 years. 2011. Available at: https://www.nap.edu/read/13150/chapter/6. Accessed April 1, 2018.

5. U.S. Food and Drug Administration. The 510(k) program: evaluating substantial equivalence in premarket notifications. 2014. Available at: http://www.fda.gov/downloads/MedicalDevices/DeviceRegulationandGuidance/GuidanceDocuments/UCM284443.pdf. Accessed April 1, 2018.

6. U.S. Food and Drug Administration. Premarket Approval (PMA). 2018. Available at: https://www.fda.gov/medicaldevices/deviceregulationandguidance/howtomarketyourdevice/premarketsubmissions/premarketapprovalpma/. Accessed April 1, 2018.

7. U.S. Food and Drug Administration. Humanitarian device exemption. 2018. Available at: https://www.fda.gov/medicaldevices/deviceregulationandguidance/howtomarketyourdevice/premarketsubmissions/humanitariandeviceexemption/default.htm. Accessed April 1, 2018.

8. U.S. Food and Drug Administration. Listing of CDRH Humanitarian Device Exemptions. 2018. Available at: https://www.fda.gov/MedicalDevices/Products

andMedicalProcedures/DeviceApprovalsandClearances/HDEApprovals/ucm16 1827.htm. Accessed April 1, 2018.

9. U.S. Food and Drug Administration. The least burdensome provisions: concept and principles. Draft guidance for industry and food and drug administration staff. 2017. Available at: https://www.fda.gov/downloads/MedicalDevices/DeviceReg ulationandGuidance/GuidanceDocuments/UCM588914.pdf. Accessed April 1, 2018.

10. Zuckerman D, Brown P, Das A. Lack of publicly available scientific evidence on the safety and effectiveness of implanted medical devices. JAMA Intern Med 2014;174(11):1781–7.

11. Rathi VK, Gadkaree SK, Ross JS, et al. US Food and Drug Administration Clearance of Moderate-Risk Otolaryngologic Devices via the 510(k) Process, 1997-2016. Otolaryngol Head Neck Surg 2017;157(4):608–17.

12. Hwang TJ, Kesselheim AS, Bourgeois FT. Postmarketing trials and pediatric device approvals. Pediatrics 2014;133(5):e1197–202.

13. Dhruva SS, Bero LA, Redberg RF. Strength of study evidence examined by the FDA in premarket approval of cardiovascular devices. JAMA 2009;302(24):2679–85.

14. Chen CE, Dhruva SS, Redberg RF. Inclusion of comparative effectiveness data in high-risk cardiovascular device studies at the time of premarket approval. JAMA 2012;308(17):1740–2.

15. Rathi VK, Wang B, Ross JS, et al. Clinical evidence supporting US Food and Drug Administration Premarket approval of high-risk otolaryngologic devices, 2000-2014. Otolaryngol Head Neck Surg 2017;156(2):285–8.

16. Hwang TJ, Sokolov E, Franklin JM, et al. Comparison of rates of safety issues and reporting of trial outcomes for medical devices approved in the European Union and United States: cohort study. BMJ 2016;353:i3323.

17. Kramer DB, Xu S, Kesselheim AS. Regulation of medical devices in the United States and European Union. N Engl J Med 2012;366(9):848–55.

18. Ardaugh BM, Graves SE, Redberg RF. The 510(k) ancestry of a metal-on-metal hip implant. N Engl J Med 2013;368(2):97–100.

19. Jacoby VL, Subak L, Waetjen LE. The FDA and the Vaginal Mesh Controversy–Further Impetus to Change the 510(k) Pathway for Medical Device Approval. JAMA Intern Med 2016;176(2):277–8.

20. Hauser RG. Here we go again–another failure of postmarketing device surveillance. N Engl J Med 2012;366(10):873–5.

21. Hines JZ, Lurie P, Yu E, et al. Left to their own devices: breakdowns in United States medical device premarket review. PLoS Med 2010;7(7):e1000280.

22. U.S. Food and Drug Administration. 510(k) Premarket Notification for Relieva Sinus Balloon Dilation Catheter. 2005. Available at: http://www.accessdata.fda.gov/cdrh_docs/pdf4/K043527.pdf. Accessed April 1, 2008.

23. U.S. Food and Drug Administration. 522 Postmarket Surveillance Study Status: Hummingbird tympanostomy tube system. 2018. Available at: https://www.fda.gov/AboutFDA/CentersOffices/OfficeofMedicalProductsandTobacco/CDRH/CD RHTransparency/ucm240318.htm. Accessed April 23, 2018.

24. Rathi VK, Kesselheim AS, Ross JS. The US Food and Drug Administration 515 Program Initiative: addressing the evidence gap for widely used, high-risk cardiovascular devices? JAMA Cardiol 2016;1(2):117–8.

25. Chatterjee S, Herrmann HC, Wilensky RL, et al. Safety and procedural success of left atrial appendage exclusion with the lariat device: a systematic review of

published reports and analytic review of the FDA MAUDE database. JAMA Intern Med 2015;175(7):1104–9.

26. Challoner D, Vodra WW. Medical devices and health–creating a new regulatory framework for moderate-risk devices. N Engl J Med 2011;365(11):977–9.

27. Garber AM. Modernizing device regulation. N Engl J Med 2010;362(13):1161–3.

28. Gottieb S, Shuren J. New steps to facilitate beneficial medical device innovation. 2017. Available at: https://blogs.fda.gov/fdavoice/index.php/tag/new-pre-and-post-market-evaluation-system-nest/. Accessed April 29, 2018.

29. Phillips PJ. Sufficiency of information in 510(k) summaries. JAMA Intern Med 2015;175(5):863–4.

30. U.S. Food and Drug Administration. Investigational device exemptions (IDEs) for early feasibility medical device clinical studies, including certain first in human (FIH) studies: guidance for industry and FDA staff. 2013. Available at: https://www.fda.gov/downloads/medicaldevices/deviceregulationandguidance/guidancedocuments/ucm279103.pdf. Accessed April 1, 2018.

31. U.S. Food and Drug Administration. Design considerations for pivotal clinical investigations for medical devices: guidance for industry, clinical investigators, institutional review boards and FDA staff. 2013. Available at: https://www.fda.gov/downloads/MedicalDevices/DeviceRegulationandGuidance/GuidanceDocuments/UCM373766.pdf. Accessed April 1, 2018.

32. Downing NS, Aminawung JA, Shah ND, et al. Clinical trial evidence supporting FDA approval of novel therapeutic agents, 2005-2012. JAMA 2014;311(4):368–77.

33. Faris O, Shuren J. An FDA viewpoint on unique considerations for medical-device clinical trials. N Engl J Med 2017;376(14):1350–7.

34. Dhruva SS, Mazure CM, Ross JS, et al. Inclusion of demographic-specific information in studies supporting US Food & Drug Administration approval of high-risk medical devices. JAMA Intern Med 2017;177(9):1390–1.

35. U.S. Food and Drug Administration. FDA action plan to enhance the collection and availability of demographic subgroup data. 2014. Available at: https://www.fda.gov/downloads/regulatoryinformation/legislation/significantamendmentstothefdcact/fdasia/ucm410474.pdf. Accessed April 1, 2018.

36. U.S. Food and Drug Administration. PMA Supplements and Amendments. 2018. Available at: https://www.fda.gov/MedicalDevices/DeviceRegulationandGuidance/HowtoMarketYourDevice/PremarketSubmissions/PremarketApprovalPMA/ucm050467.htm. Accessed April 1, 2018.

37. Rome BN, Kramer DB, Kesselheim AS. FDA approval of cardiac implantable electronic devices via original and supplement premarket approval pathways, 1979-2012. JAMA 2014;311(4):385–91.

38. Rathi VK, Ross JS, Samuel AM, et al. Postmarket modifications of high-risk therapeutic devices in otolaryngology cleared by the US Food and Drug Administration. Otolaryngol Head Neck Surg 2015;153(3):400–8.

39. Samuel AM, Rathi VK, Grauer JN, et al. How do orthopaedic devices change after their initial FDA premarket approval? Clin Orthop 2016;474(4):1053–68.

40. Zheng SY, Redberg RF. Premarket approval supplement pathway: do we know what we are getting? Ann Intern Med 2014;160(11):798–9.

41. Hildrew DM, Molony TB. Nucleus N5 CI500 series implant recall: hard failure rate at a major Cochlear implantation center. Laryngoscope 2013;123(11):2829–33.

42. Arnold W, Bredberg G, Gstöttner W, et al. Meningitis following cochlear implantation: pathomechanisms, clinical symptoms, conservative and surgical treatments. ORL J Otorhinolaryngol Relat Spec 2002;64(6):382–9.

43. U.S. Food and Drug Administration. Balancing premarket and postmarket data collection for devices subject to premarket approval: guidance for industry and food and drug administration staff. 2015. Available at: https://www.fda.gov/downloads/MedicalDevices/DeviceRegulationandGuidance/GuidanceDocuments/UCM393994.pdf. Accessed April 1, 2018.

44. Shuren J, Califf RM. Need for a national evaluation system for health technology. JAMA 2016;316(11):1153–4.

45. U.S. Food and Drug Administration. Mandatory reporting requirements: manufacturers, importers and device user facilities. 2018. Available at: https://www.fda.gov/MedicalDevices/DeviceRegulationandGuidance/PostmarketRequirements/ReportingAdverseEvents/ucm2005737.htm. Accessed April 14, 2018.

46. U.S. Food and Drug Administration. MedSun: Medical product safety network. 2018. Available at: https://www.fda.gov/MedicalDevices/Safety/MedSunMedicalProductSafetyNetwork/default.htm?source=govdelivery. Accessed April 14, 2018.

47. Engleman D, Rich S, Powell T, et al. Medical Product Safety Network (MedSun) Collaborates with medical product users to create specialty subnetworks. In: Henriksen K, Battles JB, Keyes MA, et al, editors. Advances in patient safety: new directions and alternative approaches, vol. 1: Assessment. Rockville (MD): Agency for Healthcare Research and Quality; 2008. p. 1–12.

48. U.S. Food and Drug Administration. MedWatch: The FDA Safety Information and Adverse Event Reporting Program. 2018. Available at: https://www.fda.gov/Safety/MedWatch/. Accessed April 14, 2018.

49. U.S. Food and Drug Administration. MAUDE - Manufacturer and User Facility Device Experience. 2018. Available at: https://www.accessdata.fda.gov/scripts/cdrh/cfdocs/cfMAUDE/TextSearch.cfm. Accessed April 14, 2018.

50. Woerdeman PA, Cochrane DD. Disruption of silicone valve housing in a Codman Hakim Precision valve with integrated Siphonguard. J Neurosurg Pediatr 2014; 13(5):532–5.

51. Rajan PV, Kramer DB, Kesselheim AS. Medical device postapproval safety monitoring: where does the United States stand? Circ Cardiovasc Qual Outcomes 2015;8(1):124–31.

52. Coelho DH, Tampio AJ. The utility of the MAUDE database for osseointegrated auditory implants. Ann Otol Rhinol Laryngol 2017;126(1):61–6.

53. Tambyraja RR, Gutman MA, Megerian CA. Cochlear implant complications: utility of federal database in systematic analysis. Arch Otolaryngol Head Neck Surg 2005;131(3):245–50.

54. Lenzer J, Brownlee S. Why the FDA can't protect the public. BMJ 2010;341: c4753.

55. U.S. Food and Drug Administration. 522 Postmarket Surveillance Studies – Frequently Asked Questions (FAQs). 2018. Available at: https://www.fda.gov/MedicalDevices/DeviceRegulationandGuidance/PostmarketRequirements/PostmarketSurveillance/ucm134497.htm. Accessed April 28, 2018.

56. U.S. Government Accountability Office. FDA ordered postmarket studies to better understand safety issues, and many studies are ongoing. 2015. Available at: http://www.gao.gov/assets/680/672860.pdf. Accessed April 28, 2018.

57. Rising JP, Reynolds IS, Sedrakyan A. Delays and difficulties in assessing metal-on-metal hip implants. N Engl J Med 2012;367(1):e1.

58. U.S. Food and Drug Administration. Procedures for Handling Post-Approval Studies Imposed by PMA Order. 2009. Available at: https://www.fda.gov/MedicalDevices/ucm070974.htm. Accessed April 28, 2018.

59. U.S. Food and Drug Administration. Summary of safety and effectiveness data: inspire upper airway stimulation. 2014. Available at: https://www.accessdata.fda.gov/cdrh_docs/pdf13/P130008B.pdf. Accessed April 28, 2018.

60. U.S. Food and Drug Administration. Premarket approval order: inspire upper airway stimulation. 2014. Available at: https://www.accessdata.fda.gov/cdrh_docs/pdf13/P130008A.pdf. Accessed April 28, 2018.

61. Reynolds IS, Rising JP, Coukell AJ, et al. Assessing the safety and effectiveness of devices after US Food and Drug Administration approval: FDA-mandated post-approval studies. JAMA Intern Med 2014;174(11):1773–9.

62. Wimmer NJ, Robbins S, Ssemaganda H, et al. Assessing the cost burden of United States FDA-mandated post-approval studies for medical devices. J Health Care Finance 2016;2016(Spec Features) [pii:http://www.healthfinancejournal.com/~junland/index.php/johcf/article/view/82/83].

63. Rathi VK, Krumholz HM, Masoudi FA, et al. Characteristics of clinical studies conducted over the total product life cycle of high-risk therapeutic medical devices receiving FDA premarket approval in 2010 and 2011. JAMA 2015;314(6):604–12.

64. Rathi VK. Clinical studies conducted over the total product life cycle of high-risk therapeutic medical devices receiving US Food and Drug Administration Premarket Approval in 2010 and 2011 [doctorate thesis]. New Haven (CT): Yale University; 2016.

65. Denneny JC. Regent: a new otolaryngology clinical data registry. Otolaryngol Head Neck Surg 2016;155(1):5.

Simulation Saves the Day (and Patient)

Ellen S. Deutsch, MD, MS[a,b,c,]*, Mary D. Patterson, MD, MEd[d]

KEYWORDS

- Simulation • System improvement • System engineering • Organizational resilience
- Health care education • Patient safety

KEY POINTS

- Simulation has been proved to improve the skills of individuals and the skills of teams.
- Simulation can be helpful for novices learning new skills and experienced surgeons learning new techniques and technologies.
- Simulation conducted in situ, using real teams and real equipment in real settings, can be used to evaluate and improve the safety of health care systems.

You are called to the Emergency Department (ED) to care for a 6-year-old boy with active posttonsillectomy hemorrhage. The ED team springs into action. You request suction, and a clamp and gauze, as well as directing the nurse to infuse fluids, obtain a phlebotomy specimen to type and crossmatch blood, and call the operating room (OR) to let them know you'll need to use the open trauma OR.

Fortunately, this was a simulation. The scenario for this simulation is based on actual simulations that have taken place in situ, in real EDs, with real doctors, nurses, and additional personnel participating in their actual clinical roles (eg, the ED physician participated as an ED physician) using real equipment.[1] Only the patient and the initial circumstances were simulated.

A debriefing led by a skilled facilitator immediately followed the simulation. The debriefing addressed both the actions of team members, such as task allocation and communication, and the resources and capabilities of the ED environment. Examples of resource limitations included lack of availability of the difficult airway equipment, inability of the nurse to observe the vital signs monitor, and lack of provision for family presence.[1]

Conflict of Interest: None.
[a] Pennsylvania Patient Safety Authority, 333 Market Street, Harrisburg, PA 17101, USA; [b] ECRI Institute, 5200 Butler Pike, Plymouth Meeting, PA 19462, USA; [c] Department of Anesthesiology and Critical Care, University of Pennsylvania Perelman School of Medicine, 3400 Spruce Street, Philadelphia, PA 19104, USA; [d] Department of Emergency Medicine, Center for Experiential Learning and Simulation, University of Florida, 1104 Newell Drive, Suite 445, Gainesville, FL 32610, USA
* Corresponding author. 5200 Butler Pike, Plymouth Meeting, PA 19462.
E-mail address: edeutsch@ecri.org

Following a series of simulations and debriefings, several patient care processes were modified, staffing responsibilities were adjusted, and equipment availability was modified.

And then, 2 weeks later...

You are called to the ED to care for a 6-year-old boy with active post-tonsillectomy hemorrhage. The ED team springs into action. You request suction, and a clamp and gauze, as well as directing the nurse to infuse fluids, obtain a phlebotomy specimen to type and crossmatch blood, and call the OR to let them know you'll need to use the open trauma OR.

Again, a debriefing led by a skilled facilitator immediately followed the simulation. Again, the discussion addressed the responses of the participants and the resources of the environment. Overall, the teams' response to the emergency was improved. Some of the latent safety threats previously identified had been corrected. However, some of the interventions mitigated one problem while creating others, so additional follow-up and iterative improvements will be necessary.[1]

Although this case is synthetic, each of the management details and latent safety threats described has been documented in actual simulations. Simulations, including debriefings, contain a wealth of information and opportunities to reinforce correct actions and improve patient care capabilities.

SIMULATION TO IMPROVE THE SKILLS OF INDIVIDUALS

Simulation to enhance the skills of individuals is easily understood by surgeons. Tomkins wrote about his experience saving the life of a patient with supraglottic edema, oxygen desaturation, and impending complete airway obstruction. He successfully secured the patient's airway and then, after the adrenaline surge subsided, reflected about how he had developed the skills necessary to save this patient's life by performing a rare procedure that he had never performed or seen performed on a real patient. He attributed his skills and muscle memory to practice during simulations.[2]

A variety of skills for individuals may be practiced using simulators, including controlling epistaxis; inserting myringotomy tubes; performing mastoidectomy; airway endoscopy; removal of foreign bodies from the ear canal, pharynx, esophagus or airway; sinus surgery; tracheotomy; thyroplasty; and so on. Nontechnical skills may also be practiced, such as learning how to obtain informed consent or "delivering bad news," which involves presenting distressing or unpleasant information to a simulated patient or family members. Depending on the simulation, faculty may provide ongoing coaching and feedback, or there might be a more formal debriefing as the conclusion of the simulation.

There is a growing body of evidence that simulation is an effective learning modality for individual skill development.[3–6] Individual skill development can be viewed as continuums; structured graduated progressions in skill development have been described by Kirkpatrick and by McGaghie and colleagues. Kirkpatrick[7] articulates 4 levels of learning: level 1 is reaction, a self-assessment of how participants feel about an educational program. Level 2 is learning, which includes objective measurements of skill or knowledge. Level 3 is behavior; when adapted for simulation, this is a measure of whether the learning during simulation changed the participants' actions during actual patient care. Level 4 addresses results, such as whether actual patients have better outcomes.

McGaghie and colleagues[8] present a different construct that considers levels of skill improvement as translational outcomes of simulation-based mastery learning. Level T1 is skill improvement in educational (simulation) settings; T2 is improvement in patient care practices; T3 is improvement in patient outcomes; and T4 is collateral improvements (eg, dissemination of improvements beyond the individuals who participated directly in the simulations).

Much of the literature concerning the effect of simulation on skill improvement is at the level of learner satisfaction and self-perceived improvement (eg, Kirpatrick's level 1), but there are examples of simulation improving patient outcomes in obstetrics, ophthalmology, general surgery, and critical care.[9–11] Notably, specific skills relevant to otolaryngology have been demonstrated to be transferrable from simulation to procedures on actual patients ("in vivo").[4,12] Residents trained on an endoscopic sinus surgery simulator, when compared with controls, demonstrated decreased completion time, increased confidence, and fewer technical errors on basic surgical tasks done on patients.[4] These studies have raised the question of dose response and the optimal exposure to simulation training with respect to technical performance and clinical outcomes.

Often learners participate in formative simulations, in which they are encouraged to explore, question, and try new techniques. Simulations can also be summative, including tests to formally evaluate the specific skills of individual learners. Ishman and colleagues[13] developed an objective-structured assessment of technical skills for direct laryngoscopy and rigid bronchoscopy, which consisted of task-specific evaluations (eg, selects and assembles appropriate equipment) and global evaluations (eg, instrument handling, respect for tissue). There is some evidence that global evaluations alone may provide a sufficient assessment of learner skill.[14]

SIMULATION TO IMPROVE THE SKILLS OF TEAMS

Many surgeons have participated in simulations to enhance team skills, sometimes called crew (or crisis) resource management or simply team training. Skills practiced may include leadership, communication, team coordination, and resource allocation. Often these simulations are staged as "scenarios," which include diagnosing and then treating a simulated patient's medical condition, such as hemorrhage following transoral robotic resection of malignancy, rapidly expanding neck hematoma following thyroid surgery, airway obstruction from angioedema, and management of a tracheotomy tube in a false passage. The same high-technology infant simulator that can be used as a "task trainer" to help learners develop skills in removing aspirated foreign bodies can be placed in a patient care context that requires teamwork for optimal management. A simulated nurse and anesthesiologist may also participate, so that the learner must accomplish more than the psychomotor skill of removing the foreign body; the learner must also coordinate with the team to ensure that the patient remains adequately anesthetized and ventilated during the foreign body removal procedure. If a high-technology manikin is used, the manikin's vital signs can be displayed on a patient care monitor, on which desaturation or other conditions occur in real time. Some manikins can demonstrate asymmetric chest wall motion with "breathing," stridor and laryngospasm (eg, the vocal folds come together).

Although simulation is often used for training students and residents, it has the potential application for otolaryngologists at any level of experience who desire to learn new techniques or take advantage of new technologies, as well as otolaryngologists who desire to refresh skills following a hiatus in the use of those skills. It also serves as an ongoing means to learn or refresh critical communication and teamwork skills.

Simulation debriefings are key to learning and may take longer than the patient care component of the simulation. Debriefings often focus first, on the teamwork aspects of the stimulation, and then address the medical management. It is important to help learners understand what they did well as well as processes they might improve.[15] Expert facilitators guide learners to recognize correct decisions and actions, as well as gaps in performance, and to develop and articulate their own lessons.

SIMULATION TO IMPROVE SYSTEMS

The next frontier for simulation is the use of simulation to improve health care systems, and this use of simulation may have the greatest impact on patient safety. Simulation can be used to improve the systems we work within, around, because of, and despite. Health care is more than complicated; health care is a complex adaptive system, which means, among other things, that the structure and interactions of the components of health care are so complex that they can never be completely knowable.[16] Simulation can be used to expose aspects of patient care delivery that are not necessarily evident prospectively, during planning, or retrospectively, during investigations or audits. Actual patient care processes may become most evident during simulations conducted "in situ" using real teams and real equipment, in actual patient care locations. Simulation can help move the understanding of patient care processes from "work as imagined" closer to the reality of "work as done."[17] In situ simulation allows the examination of how work is accomplished in sanctioned and unsanctioned ways in order to care for the patient. In particular, in situ simulation facilitates a better understanding of the constraints and workarounds that exist in a system as well as the adaptive capacity of the individuals working within the system and therefore of the system itself. This aspect of simulation aligns with Safety II and demonstrates how simulation provides a window on"normal" work and how "normal work" succeeds.[17]

One of the most popular models of the components of health care systems is the SEIPS model. In this model, Holden and colleagues[18] describe complex relationships between the following components of the health care work system: persons (patients and providers); tasks; technology and tools; organization; processes; and outcomes at the level of the patient, the employee, and the organization. In reality, the capabilities of individuals, teams, and the environment are inseparable; and the outcomes of actual patient care involve complex interactions among the patient, the care providers, and the environment, but it can be a useful conceptual construct to look at the environment that surrounds the provider or the team of providers. As in the example at the beginning of this article, simulation can be used in an iterative fashion to explore, understand, and modify many aspects of the work environment. Simulation can be used proactively, such as while planning a new patient care area to fine-tune the room layout or the location of tools and equipment or before implementing a new patient care process, to ensure that all of the necessary resources are in place. Simulation can be used to help prepare office staff for patient care emergencies or unplanned computer down-time.

Simpao and colleagues[19] and the Center for Simulation, Advanced Education and Innovation at the Children's Hospital of Philadelphia have used simulation to prepare for the unusual surgical procedure of separating conjoined twins. Weintraub and colleagues[20] simulated concurrent care of an anesthetized (simulated) patient while maintaining documentation in the electronic health record (EHR) to help prepare providers for the implementation of a new EHR module. Simulation can also be used after a serious patient care event, as a component of a retrospective analysis, in a forensic manner.

Whether simulations are used in a reactive manner or in a proactive manner such as for system improvement, debriefing remains essential to support individual, team, and organizational learning, but the focus of the discussion shifts to the relationships between the care providers and the care environment. Debriefing using a system perspective based on Safety II principles would emphasize understanding and reinforcing "what went well"[17] as well as what could be improved.

These examples speak to the ways in which simulation is a useful technique for Resilience Engineering. Resilience Engineering, at its core, involves 4 activities: monitoring, learning, responding, and anticipating.[21] Simulation allows managers and frontline workers to monitor the adaptive capacity of the system (through simulation exercises) and to practice ways to respond to perturbations in the system. It also provides a means to anticipate and practice for the unexpected, even when as described previously, individuals may not have experienced a particular situation in actual clinical practice.

Perhaps most importantly, simulation has the potential to "enhance the repertoire of responses" to a disruptive event in the system.[22] Wears and Morrison posit that system's experiences with disruptive events that are associated with appropriate feedback and coaching may actually improve the ways in which the individuals within the system are able to manage such disruptions.

> *"This contributes to building "margin" - a collection of informal buffers, resources, short-cuts, tradeoffs and procedures - a "bag of tricks" - that can be called on in either impromptu or extemporaneous ways. We postulate that resilient systems are characterized by their skill at capturing and learning from these experiences; which, paradoxically, may be dependent on their relatively frequently experiencing them."[22]*

The irony of course is that when disruptive events occur in the actual clinical system, it may result in delays in care, morbidity, and even mortality. Simulation provides the opportunity to practice the response to unusual and disruptive events and receive the appropriate feedback as often as desired. In turn, this results in building margin and adaptive capacity in the system—the "bag of tricks" that the team can use when unexpected or when disruptive events occur. In this way simulation provides a means to facilitate the development of resilience in the system.

SIMULATORS

Simulation construction is based on developing the desired learning objectives and then incorporating simulators that deliver the appropriate cues. There is a wide range of possible simulators, depending on the objectives of the educational experience. These may include manikin-type simulators, task trainers, virtual reality, box trainers, cadavers, biological tissue (eg, pig's feet), and anesthetized animals. Simulators may replicate whole patients or anatomic parts of patients (eg, an intubation head). "Standardized patients" are actors, trained to provide scripted interactions with learners and then provide feedback and/or evaluations of the learners.

Contemporary simulators may incorporate technology that allows responses to interventions, such as oxygen desaturation if the manikin is not ventilated, as well as technology that can track and provide feedback and/or data about the user's actions, such as time spent, aliquots of topical anesthetic administered, or appropriate and inappropriate intersections with specific anatomic areas (eg, drilling into the dura). Contemporary manufacturing methods, such as 3-dimensional printing, allow the replication of patient-specific anatomy. There are virtual reality and augmented reality otolaryngology simulators under development or commercially available, and the number and sophistication of simulators is rapidly evolving.

On the other hand, there are simple simulators and task trainers that are homemade, or inexpensive, that have great fidelity for the desired task. The simulator for the separation of conjoined twins was designed to allow the operative team to anticipate how the ventilator and intravenous line tubing should be organized so that each twin would have their own resources without entanglement or contamination once the twins were separated. The simulator consisted of 2 dolls sewn together, low tech but effective. Simulators may include cardboard parts, gelatin, rubber bands, eggs, bone wax, and a variety of other objects, which may still provide a foundation for appropriate skill development. In simulation, the attributes of technology, fidelity, and cost have nonlinear relationships.

There are, of course, limitations to simulation. Implementation can be labor intensive, and some simulation-based educational processes are difficult to scale. Debriefing requires training, skill, and ongoing practice. There is a risk of discrepant modeling, with inaccurate representations of physical findings or inaccurate timing or duration of events (eg, the deterioration of a patient during a simulation may occur faster or slower than it would occur during actual patient care). In particular, Otolaryngology is a relatively small market, so the physical features in commercially available simulators are not always finessed to the degree of accuracy desired. None-the-less, simulation offers an opportunity to practice or explore events and circumstances that affect patient safety, selected because of their interest to the participants, occurring at the relative convenience of the participants, without direct risks to real patients.[23,24]

SUMMARY

Simulation can be used to improve patient safety by improving health care delivery processes as well as the skills of individuals and teams. Health care delivery is a complex adaptive system, which can never be completely knowable, but simulation can expose system hazards and strengths, to move our understanding from "work as imagined" closer to "work as done." Simulation used to explore and iteratively improve the safety of patient care processes is a powerful tool.

REFERENCES

1. Geis GL, Pio B, Pendergrass TL, et al. Simulation to assess the safety of new health-care teams and new facilities. Simul Healthc 2011;6(3):125–33.
2. Tompkins JJ. Use of simulation boot camps to train junior otolaryngology residents: A resident's testimonial. JAMA Otolaryngol Head Neck Surg 2014;140(5):1–2.
3. Wiet GJ, Stredney D, Kerwin T, et al. Virtual temporal bone dissection system: OSU virtual temporal bone system: development and testing. Laryngoscope 2012;122(Suppl 1):S1–12.
4. Fried MP, Sadoughi B, Gibber MJ, et al. From virtual reality to the operating room: The endoscopic sinus surgery simulator experiment. Otolaryngol Head Neck Surg 2010;142(2):202–7.
5. McGaghie WC, Issenberg SB, Cohen ER, et al. Does simulation-based medical education with deliberate practice yield better results than traditional clinical education? A meta-analytic comparative review of the evidence. Acad Med 2011; 86(6):706–11.
6. Cook DA. How much evidence does it take? A cumulative meta-analysis of outcomes of simulation-based education. Med Educ 2014;48(8):750–60.
7. Kirkpatrick D. Great ideas revisited. Training and development 1996;50(1):54.
8. McGaghie WC, Issenberg SB, Barsuk JH, et al. A critical review of simulation-based mastery learning with translational outcomes. Med Educ 2014;48:375–85.
9. Draycott TJ, Crofts JF, Ash JP, et al. Improving neonatal outcome through practical shoulder dystocia training. Obstet Gynecol 2008;112(1):14–20.

10. Wolfe H, Zebuhr C, Topjian AA, et al. Interdisciplinary ICU cardiac arrest debriefing improves survival outcomes. Crit Care Med 2014;42(7):1688–95.
11. Cox T, Seymour N, Stefanidis D. Moving the needle: Simulation's impact on patient outcomes [review]. Surg Clin North Am 2015;95(4):827–38.
12. Howells TH, Emery FM, Twentyman JE. Endotracheal intubation training using a simulator. an evaluation of the laerdal adult intubation model in the teaching of endotracheal intubation. Br J Anaesth 1973;45(4):400–2.
13. Ishman SL, Benke JR, Johnson K, et al. Blinded evaluation of interrater reliability of an operative competency assessment tool for direct laryngoscopy and rigid bronchoscopy. Arch Otolaryngol Head Neck Surg 2012;138(10):916–22.
14. Regehr G, MacRae H, Reznick RK, et al. Comparing the psychometric properties of checklists and global rating scales for assessing performance on an OSCE-format examination. Acad Med 1998;73(9):993–7.
15. Ellis S, Davidi I. After-event reviews: Drawing lessons from successful and failed experience. J Appl Psychol 2005;90(5):857–71.
16. Braithwaite J, Clay-Williams R, Nugus P, et al. Health care as a complex adaptive system. In: Hollnagel E, Braithwaite J, Wears RL, editors. Resilient health care. Farnham (England): Ashgate; 2013. p. 57–76.
17. Hollnagel E, Wears R, Braithwaite J. From safety-I to safety-II: a white paper. The resilient health care net. Published by the University of Southern Denmark, University of Florida, USA, and Macquarie University, Australia. 2015.
18. Holden RJ, Carayon P, Gurses AP, et al. SEIPS 2.0: A human factors framework for studying and improving the work of healthcare professionals and patients. Ergonomics 2013;56(11):1669–86.
19. Simpao AF, Wong R, Ferrara TJ, et al. From simulation to separation surgery: a tale of two twins. Anesthesiology 2014;120(1):110.
20. Weintraub AY, Deutsch ES, Hales RL, et al. Using high-technology simulators to prepare anesthesia providers before implementation of a new electronic health record module: a technical report. Anesth Analg 2017;124(6):1815–9.
21. Fairbanks RJ, Wears RL, Woods DD, et al. Resilience and resilience engineering in health care. Jt Comm J Qual Patient Saf 2014;40(8):376–83.
22. Wears RL, Morrison B. Levels of resilience: Moving from resilience to resilience engineering. Proceedings from the 5th symposium on resilience engineering, managing trade-offs. Sophia Antipolis (France): Resilience Engineering Association; 2013.
23. Deutsch ES. Simulation in otolaryngology: Smart dummies and more. Otolaryngol Head Neck Surg 2011;145(6):899–903.
24. Kneebone R. Simulation in surgical training: Educational issues and practical implications. Med Educ 2003;37(3):267–77.

Clinical Indices to Drive Quality Improvement in Otolaryngology

Christine L. Barron, BA[a], Charles A. Elmaraghy, MD[b,c],
Stephanie Lemle, MBA[d], Wallace Crandall, MD, MMM[d,e],
Richard J. Brilli, MD[f], Kris R. Jatana, MD[b,c,*]

KEYWORDS

- Index • Indices • Pediatric • Tracheostomy • Tracheotomy • Quality improvement

KEY POINTS

- Care indices are valuable tools for standardizing, quantifying, and monitoring the reliability and documentation of care provided to complex patient populations.
- Outside of the authors' initial work, there is currently no published literature using care indices to assess outcomes in otolaryngology.
- The authors developed a Pediatric Tracheostomy Care Index (PTCI) to drive quality improvement efforts at their institution, comprised of 9 elements deemed essential for safe care of children with a tracheostomy tube. They believe this PTCI is broadly generalizable.
- Within the PTCI, focused quality improvement projects can be performed to target challenging elements, such as the elimination of advanced stage postoperative tracheostomy–related pressure wounds, which has been maintained at the authors' institution for 5 consecutive years.

Disclosure Statement: K.R. Jatana serves as a product safety medical consultant for Intertek Product Intelligence Group, Inc; K.R. Jatana and C.A. Elmaraghy receive royalties for a novel patented tracheostomy tube collar, known as Comfort Collar, licensed to Marpac Inc; C.A. Elmaraghy serves as a consultant to Smith and Nephew, Inc. There are no further disclosures among the authors.
^a The Ohio State University College of Medicine, 370 West 9th Avenue, Columbus, OH 43210, USA; ^b Department of Pediatric Otolaryngology, Nationwide Children's Hospital, 555 South 18th Street, Suite 2A, Columbus, OH 43205, USA; ^c Department of Otolaryngology-Head and Neck Surgery, Wexner Medical Center at Ohio State University, 915 Olentangy River Road, Columbus, OH 43212, USA; ^d Quality Improvement Services, Nationwide Children's Hospital, 700 Children's Drive, Suite 2A, Columbus, OH 43205, USA; ^e Division of Pediatric Gastroenterology, Hepatology, and Nutrition, Department of Pediatrics, Ohio State University College of Medicine, Nationwide Children's Hospital, 700 Children's Drive, Columbus, OH 43205, USA; ^f Division of Pediatric Critical Care Medicine, Department of Pediatrics, Ohio State University College of Medicine, Nationwide Children's Hospital, 700 Children's Drive, Columbus, OH 43205, USA
* Corresponding author. Department of Pediatric Otolaryngology, Nationwide Children's Hospital, 555 South 18th Street, Suite 2A, Columbus, OH 43205.
E-mail address: Kris.Jatana@nationwidechildrens.org

Otolaryngol Clin N Am 52 (2019) 123–133
https://doi.org/10.1016/j.otc.2018.08.008
0030-6665/19/© 2018 Elsevier Inc. All rights reserved.

INTRODUCTION

Tracheostomy procedures in young children account for a substantial proportion of adverse events in pediatric otolaryngology.[1] Pediatric tracheostomy patients represent a complex and heterogeneous group with multiple comorbid conditions. Thus, effective care requires intensive, multidisciplinary collaboration from a variety of stakeholders spanning multiple medical specialties and ancillary services. Currently, there is both ample opportunity and widely recognized need for quality improvement in pediatric tracheostomy care.[2] In this article, the authors describe the use of a patient safety index that both defines optimal care and serves as a clinical management tool to improve performance across the continuum of tracheostomy care.

In 2010, the authors' hospital introduced the Preventable Harm Index (PHI), a novel metric that sums the total number of undesirable patient events—preventable harm plus missed opportunities to provide optimal care—within a given time frame.[3] A lower PHI value signifies fewer undesirable events and better overall program performance. Since its introduction, the index concept has been applied in multiple service lines[4] and is being used in several pediatric hospitals as a clinical management tool to maximize patient safety.[5,6] However, outside of their initial work, there is currently *no published literature* using care indices to assess outcomes in otolaryngology.

Building on the PHI framework, a Pediatric Tracheostomy Care Index (PTCI) was created to standardize tracheostomy care, monitor care provided, and focus interventions to propel quality improvement at their institution (**Fig. 1**). The PTCI comprises 9 elements deemed essential for safe care of children with a tracheostomy tube. It spans the domains of preoperative evaluation, intraoperative documentation, and guidelines for postoperative follow-up. Therefore, it is an aggregate performance metric for tracheostomy care. The authors hypothesized that implementation and measurement of

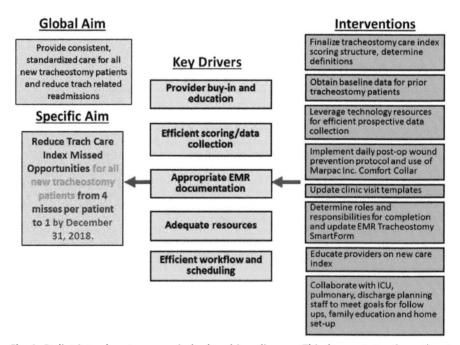

Fig. 1. Pediatric tracheostomy care index key driver diagram. This demonstrates the authors' project aim, key drivers, and defined interventions.

the PTCI, alongside targeted quality improvement initiatives, would substantially improve care reliability among their tracheostomy patients. They also present some of their focused work on prevention of post-op tracheostomy advanced stage pressure injuries, which is included as one of their PTCI measures.

METHODS

This quality improvement project was performed at a large, academic pediatric tertiary and quaternary care medical center, which serves patients in the Midwest region of the United States. Annually, the authors have more than 30,000 clinic visits per year, and perform more than 9000 surgical procedures. Clinical providers in the department of pediatric otolaryngology include 11 fellowship-trained surgeons, 1 fellow, 4 advanced practice nurses, 15 registered nurses, and 20 rotating residents during their pediatric otolaryngology training.

The PCTI score is calculated for pediatric patients getting a new tracheostomy tube placed at the authors' institution and maintaining longitudinal care for over a minimum of 12 months. Elements of the PCTI are monitored within the electronic medical record by their internal quality improvement services data team and reported on a quarterly basis to providers. A total of 42 patients were evaluated during the baseline period of January 2014 to September 2015, and an additional 61 patients were included since project initiation between October 2015 and December 2017. This project sought to create an index method for care standardization to serve as a measuring stick for the care provided over time.

Table 1	
Pediatric tracheostomy care index elements	
Elements	**Number Of Missed Events**
Preoperative	
Tracheostomy Advanced Practice Nurse consulted and teaching initiated preoperatively	n
Postoperative	
Cardiopulmonary resuscitation and emergency care training for parents	n
No tracheostomy-related pressure ulcer	n
Home equipment set up before discharge	n
Follow-up appointment scheduled before discharge	n
Complex patient EMR SmartForm (tracheostomy section) updated before discharge	n
Postdischarge	
Postoperative ENT office visit occurred within 60 d of hospital discharge	n
Emergency bag of supplies checked at first postoperative visit[a]	n
Airway visualization within 12 mo of tracheostomy placement	n
Pediatric Tracheostomy Care Index (PTCI)	Sum

[a] Emergency equipment to facilitate urgently changing the tracheostomy tube for plugging or dislodgement. It contains suction, suction catheters, suction tubing, and an identical spare and half size smaller tracheostomy tube for each patient.

The PCTI for all new tracheostomy patients was analyzed quarterly as shown in **Table 1**. All elements should have occurred in the appropriate time frame; if not, it is counted as an event and added to the PTCI. Consistent surveillance of outcomes was critical to ensure that the authors had timely, objective data to identify care areas for further intervention. Through several Plan-Do-Study-Act cycles, they identified additional interventions through feedback solicited from initiative participants. The authors' PTCI key driver diagram and implemented interventions are shown in **Fig. 1**.

Finally, a focused, multidisciplinary institutional protocol (**Table 2**) was created to address post-operative advanced stage pressure injuries (a component of the PCTI). An example of their protective dressing placed in the operating room at the time of tracheostomy tube placement is shown in **Fig. 2**. This is changed daily by the multidisciplinary rounding team, along with complete inspection of the entire circumference of the neck. The institutional review board reviewed these projects and ruled them exempt, given their quality improvement focus.

RESULTS

The PCTI was reduced by 50%, from an average of 4.30 missed care opportunities per patient during baseline period to 2.15 per patient during the intervention period, $P<.001$ (**Fig. 3**). Using a *pareto chart* (**Fig. 4**) of missed opportunities for 2017, the authors are able to focus future interventions accordingly. For example, they noted that improvement in scheduling follow-up appointments before discharge (23.9% missed) was needed. Similarly, when the clinic follow-up fails to take place (19.6%), the check for the presence of an emergency bag is also missed (19.6%). Follow-up is also critical to ensure that the annual airway evaluation is performed (19.6% of missed care opportunities). Within PTCI, there were no advanced stage posttracheostomy pressure injuries; furthermore, there have not been any in the postoperative period for greater than 5 consecutive years at the authors' institution (**Fig. 5**).

DISCUSSION

Traditionally, studies in quality improvement and patient safety report their results in terms of rates. This involves the challenging task of defining both the number of harm events (the numerator) and the number of opportunities or patients vulnerable to harm (the denominator).[7] In contrast, a care index sums only the total number of individual events—preventable harm plus missed opportunities for providing optimal care. Emphasis on the numerator makes the care index a simple, easily understood

Table 2 Nationwide Children's Hospital daily multidisciplinary rounds, postoperative pediatric tracheostomy protocol	
Rounding Team	**Daily Wound Care Regimen**
1. Otolaryngology senior resident and/or fellow 2. Certified wound care specialist 3. Bedside RN 4. Respiratory therapist	1. Collar and protective dressing removed 2. Entire neck skin integrity examined while tube stabilized by otolaryngology team 3. Neck skin cleaned and dried 4. Cavilon3M, no sting barrier film applied to skin 5. Mepilex Lite applied circumferentially 5. Placement of a new Marpac Inc Comfort Collar 6. Final positioning and sedation level reviewed

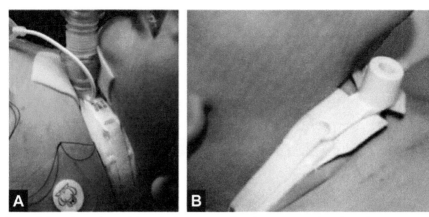

Fig. 2. (A) A circumferential neck dressing is placed at time of initial tracheostomy tube placement. This includes use of the Marpac Comfort Collar, which contains an attached/built-in neoprene dressing that directly fits under the flanges of the tube itself. (B) After initial tracheostomy tube change, the Marpac Comfort Collar is utilized for consistent skin protection under tube flanges.

metric. Because it represents the total number of undesirable events, the programmatic goal centers on driving the index toward zero; thus, it can be a highly personal and motivational tool for clinical staff. The concept focuses on not missing any essential care element for each patient.

In the nearly 20 years since the Institute of Medicine published *To Err is Human*, otolaryngology has made significant progress in quality improvement and patient safety. There now exist large, multiinstitutional survey and database studies analyzing surgical quality outcomes and identifying high-yield areas for quality improvement,[8] as

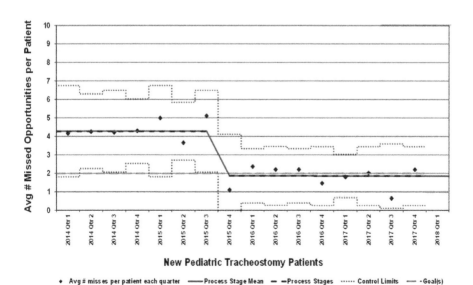

Fig. 3. Pediatric tracheostomy care index. The PTCI was reduced by 50% of missed care opportunities per patient compared with a baseline period.

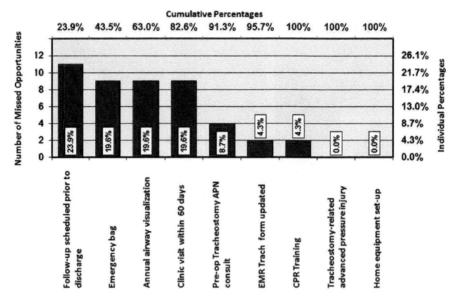

Fig. 4. Pareto chart. A breakdown of missed opportunities in 2017 helps determine future areas for targeted intervention.

well as international coalitions collaborating to define best practices for the field.[9] However, despite significant progress, relatively few studies in otolaryngology describe the implementation of clinical management tools—including clinical pathways, care bundles, checklists, and care indices—to enact quality improvement interventions at the point of care (**Table 3**).

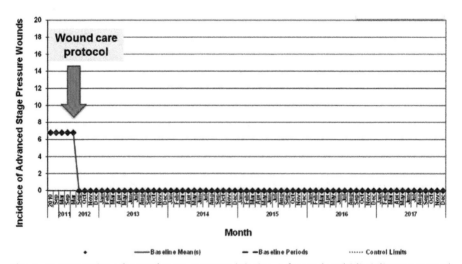

Fig. 5. Postoperative advanced stage pressure injuries. A focused multidisciplinary protocol was created to address postoperative advanced stage pressure injuries (a component of the PCTI). Since implementation, advanced stage wounds have been eliminated during the postoperative period at the authors' institution.

Table 3
Literature review (2000–2018) of clinical management tools in otolaryngology

Search Term[a]	Citations
Preventable harm index, care index, clinical index, quality index	Crandall et al,[4] 2017
Clinical care pathways, integrated care pathways, collaborative care pathways, care maps	Chen et al,[21] 2000 Gendron et al,[22] 2002 Yeuh et al,[19] 2003 Dautremont et al,[23] 2013 Yeung et al,[18] 2014 Gordon et al,[20] 2014 Yetzer et al,[14] 2017
Clinical care bundles	Hettige et al,[28] 2008 Boesch et al,[29] 2012 Visscher et al,[30] 2013 McEvoy et al,[31] 2017
Checklist, patient safety checklists	Helmiö et al,[32] 2011 Soler et al,[33] 2012

[a] In conjunction with: otolaryngology OR otorhinolaryngology OR laryngology OR audiology OR rhinology OR otology OR neurotology OR maxillofacial OR craniofacial OR hearing OR ear OR nose OR throat OR head OR neck OR tracheostomy OR tracheotomy OR wound OR pressure ulcers.

The creation of clinical management tools begins with the development of evidence-based clinical guidelines. To date, the American Academy of Otolaryngology—Head and Neck Surgery Foundation has published 14 clinical guidelines on subjects ranging from tinnitus to Bell palsy. In addition, large-scale, multiinstitutional efforts have been made to standardize protocols and provide consensus recommendations. Organizations such as the Global Tracheotomy Collaborative are collaborating to create international databases of outcomes data with the goal of establishing best practices for tracheostomy care in children and are thus working to fill a relative dearth of clinical guidelines in pediatric otolaryngology.[9] Within head and neck cancer, multiple studies examine compliance with clinical practice guidelines,[9,10] as well as the impact of protocol noncompliance on overall patient outcomes.[11–13]

The most prominent examples in otolaryngology by which clinical guidelines are translated into management tools for quality improvement can be seen in clinical pathways.[14–18] Pathways are management algorithms for specific patient populations with a predictable clinical course, in which tasks performed across multiple services are defined, optimized, and sequenced in order to standardize care delivery. Their use is most notable in head and neck surgery, as the complex, multidisciplinary care needs of these patients make this field ideal for their implementation.[19,20] Chen and colleagues[21] described implementation of a clinical pathway for management of patients undergoing postoperative unilateral neck dissection, noting decreased lengths of stay (4.0–2.0 days, $P = .001$) and median costs of care. Similarly, Gendron and colleagues[22] noted a decrease in intensive care unit lengths of stay (2.2–1.1 days, $P = .001$), median total charges, and postoperative pneumonia (12%–1%, $P = .02$) across a 3-year period in patients undergoing cancer resection. More recently, Dautremont and colleagues[23] demonstrated that patients managed using clinical pathways had fewer postdischarge encounters and lower readmission costs, whereas Yeung and colleagues[18] showed that patients participating in clinical care pathways had 32.5% fewer pulmonary complications ($P<.0001$).

Overall, care bundles are another type of tool becoming widely implemented in medicine. A bundle is a structured set of evidence-based practices that, when performed collectively, improve patient outcomes.[24] By definition, the set of interventions contained within a bundle must be implemented in its entirety; therefore, bundles serve to unify best practices and eliminate unreliable, idiosyncratic care. It has been shown that by carefully following a prevention bundle, ventilator-acquired pneumonia can be effectively eliminated[25] and central line infections significantly reduced.[26,27]

However, there are relatively few published instances of bundles being implemented in otolaryngology, all focusing on the reduction of pressure ulcers.[28–31] Boesch and colleagues[29] reported implementation of a bundle consisting of pressure ulcer risk and skin assessment, ensuring moisture-free and pressure-free device interfaces. This resulted in a decrease in the rate of patients who developed pressure ulcer (8.1%–0.3% after bundle implementation). Visscher reported use of a bundle that included additional elements focusing on education/awareness and the use of specific "champions" for monitoring and reinforcement, resulting in a significant decrease in the rate of pressure ulcers observed in the PICU (14.3/1000 patient-days to 3.7/1000 patient-days, $P<.01$).[30] Finally, McEvoy and colleagues[31] reported implementation of a multidisciplinary wound prevention protocol that was successful in the elimination of all tracheostomy-related advanced stage, hospital-acquired pressure injuries.

Finally, checklists represent another management tool intimately related to bundles and care pathways. Checklists standardize important practices across institutions and increase the likelihood that these practices occur during a particular event. Helmiö and colleagues[32] evaluated the incorporation of the WHO Surgical Safety Checklist into otolaryngology and found that the checklist improved verification of patient's identity, awareness of patient's medical history, discussion of critical events, and communication between team members. Soler and colleagues[33] applied a checklist designed specifically for endoscopic sinus surgery. Their analysis found that before checklist implementation, significant heterogeneity exists with regard to performance of specific tasks and that checklist adoption was effective at standardizing practice across institutions and increasing the performance of individual safety tasks.

To date, outside of the author's initial work, there is no published literature using care indices to assess outcomes in otolaryngology. The PCTI differs in several ways from the other implementation management tools described earlier. First, an index includes elements that span the continuum of tracheostomy care, from preoperative to postdischarge considerations. Therefore, it takes more than just a checklist of processes to carry out around a specific event. Rather, it represents all opportunities to maximize a patient's health care experience over a long-term treatment course. Whereas care pathways are predominantly limited to individual conditions and patients, care indices have the potential to measure care reliability across several conditions or health care settings.

Care indices are also fundamentally different from bundles, which must be completed in their entirety in order to realize improved clinical outcomes. Likewise, several hospitals focus on serious safety events or "never events" in their internal quality assessments. In contrast, the PCTI contains several small elements that alone may take many years' worth of data to yield meaningful results but are nevertheless essential for patient care. Although the elements are not all equally consequential, their presence raises the level of awareness among hospital staff of their importance in the care continuum. Furthermore, despite being relatively low at baseline (4.2%), the PCTI was reduced by 50%. Therefore, regardless of patient volume or illness severity, a care index can be used as a tool to improve care reliability within a system.

There are some limitations to using a care index within a health system. A clinical index, like the PCTI, is not a rate but rather based on a sum of missed care events per patient. Equal importance is given to all essential care elements for each individual patient, and the goal is to get to zero. Although rates may be easier to benchmark for comparison between institutions, a care index would require the same parameters and similar internal data collection mechanisms to be used across institutions. Finally, clinical indices require adequate infrastructure and quality improvement services required to consistently and reliably track the clinical data. In addition, the presence of an electronic medical record with data capabilities is needed to be able to efficiently extract appropriate data.

SUMMARY

To date, otolaryngology-specific clinical indices have not been widely used. However, they have the potential to standardize, quantify, and monitor care provided to patients over time. The use of the PTCI has helped identify missed opportunities and improve reliability of care provided to a complex patient population and fosters interventions to optimize patient care. In addition, other focused quality improvement projects can help further advance specific index measures, such as reduction of tracheostomy-related pressure injuries. Continued surveillance will steer future directions to provide optimal patient care and perhaps further broader utilization of care indices.

REFERENCES

1. Shah RK, Stey AM, Jatana KR, et al. Identification of opportunities for quality improvement and outcome measurement in pediatric otolaryngology. JAMA Otolaryngol Head Neck Surg 2014;140(11):1019–26.
2. Ishman SL, Hart CK. Improving outcomes and promoting quality in otolaryngology-beyond the national surgical quality improvement program. JAMA Otolaryngol Head Neck Surg 2016;142(3):247–8.
3. Brilli RJ, McClead RE, Davis T, et al. The preventable harm index: an effective motivator to facilitate the drive to zero. J Pediatr 2010;157(4):681–3.
4. Crandall W, Davis JT, Dotson J, et al. Clinical indices can standardize and monitor pediatric care: a novel mechanism to improve quality and safety. J Pediatr 2017; 193:190–5.e1.
5. Olshefski R, Vaughan M, YoungSaleme T, et al. The cancer care index: a novel metric to assess overall performance of a pediatric oncology program. J Patient Saf 2016;1–6. https://doi.org/10.1097/PTS.0000000000000267.
6. Lyren A, Brilli R, Bird M, et al. Ohio children's hospitals' solutions for patient safety: a framework for pediatric patient safety improvement. J Healthc Qual 2016;38(4): 213–22.
7. Crandall WV, Davis JT, McClead R, et al. Is preventable harm the right patient safety metric? Pediatr Clin North Am 2012;59(6):1279–92.
8. Mahida JB, Asti L, Boss EF, et al. Tracheostomy placement in children younger than 2 years: 30-day outcomes using the National Surgical Quality Improvement Program Pediatric. JAMA Otolaryngol Head Neck Surg 2016;142(3):241–6.
9. Lavin J, Shah R, Greenlick H, et al. The global tracheostomy collaborative: one institution's experience with a new quality improvement initiative. Int J Pediatr Otorhinolaryngol 2016;80:106–8.
10. Lewis CM, Hessel AC, Roberts DB, et al. Prereferral head and neck cancer treatment: compliance with national comprehensive cancer network treatment guidelines. Arch Otolaryngol Head Neck Surg 2010;136(12):1205–11.

11. Peters LJ, O'Sullivan B, Giralt J, et al. Critical impact of radiotherapy protocol compliance and quality in the treatment of advanced head and neck cancer: results from TROG 02.02. J Clin Oncol 2010;28(18):2996–3001.

12. Schwam ZG, Sosa JA, Roman S, et al. Receipt of care discordant with practice guidelines is associated with compromised overall survival in nasopharyngeal carcinoma. Clin Oncol 2016;28(6):402–9.

13. Shah BA, Qureshi MM, Jalisi S, et al. Analysis of decision making at a multidisciplinary head and neck tumor board incorporating evidence-based National Cancer Comprehensive Network (NCCN) guidelines. Pract Radiat Oncol 2016;6(4): 248–54.

14. Yetzer JG, Pirgousis P, Li Z, et al. Clinical pathway implementation improves efficiency of care in a maxillofacial head and neck surgery unit. J Oral Maxillofac Surg 2017;75(1):190–6.

15. Altman KW. Improving health outcomes and value with care pathways: the otolaryngologist's role. Otolaryngol Head Neck Surg 2014;151(4):527–9.

16. Husbands J, Weber R, Karpati R, et al. Clinical care pathways: decreasing resource utilization in head and neck surgical patients. Otolaryngol Head Neck Surg 1999;121(6):755–9. Available at: http://search.ebscohost.com/login.aspx?direct=true&db=rzh&AN=107111400&site=ehost-live.

17. Brietzke SE. Individualized clinical practice guidelines: the next step in the evidence-based health care evolution? Otolaryngol Head Neck Surg 2014; 150(3):342–5.

18. Yeung JK, Dautremont JF, Harrop AR, et al. Reduction of pulmonary complications and hospital length of stay with a clinical care pathway after head and neck reconstruction. Plast Reconstr Surg 2014;133(6):1477–84.

19. Yueh B, Weaver EM, Bradley EH, et al. A critical evaluation of critical pathways in head and neck cancer. Arch Otolaryngol Head Neck Surg 2003;129(1):89–95.

20. Gordon S. Effectiveness of critical care pathways for head and neck cancer surgery: a systematic review. Head Neck 2014;36(10):1391.

21. Chen AY, Callender D, Mansyur C, et al. The impact of clinical pathways on the practice of head and neck oncologic surgery: the University of Texas M. D. Anderson Cancer Center Experience. Arch Otolaryngol Head Neck Surg 2000; 126(3):322–6. Available at: http://www.ncbi.nlm.nih.gov/pubmed/10722004.

22. Gendron KM, Lai SY, Weinstein GS, et al. Clinical care pathway for head and neck cancer. Arch Otolaryngol Head Neck Surg 2002;128(3):258.

23. Dautremont JF, Rudmik LR, Yeung J, et al. Cost-effectiveness analysis of a postoperative clinical care pathway in head and neck surgery with microvascular reconstruction. J Otolaryngol 2013;42(1):59.

24. Haraden C. What is a bundle? Institute for Healthcare Improvement (IHI). 2018. Available at: http://www.ihi.org/resources/Pages/ImprovementStories/WhatIsaBundle.aspx. Accessed April 30, 2018.

25. Bigham MT, Amato R, Bondurrant P, et al. Ventilator-associated pneumonia in the pediatric intensive care unit: characterizing the problem and implementing a sustainable solution. J Pediatr 2009;154(4):582–7.e2.

26. Miller MR, Griswold M, Harris JM, et al. Decreasing PICU catheter-associated bloodstream infections: NACHRI's quality transformation efforts. Pediatrics 2010;125(2):206–13.

27. Miller MR, Niedner MF, Huskins WC, et al. Reducing PICU central line-associated bloodstream infections: 3-year results. Pediatrics 2011;128(5):e1077–83.

28. Hettige R, Arora A, Ifeacho S, et al. Improving tracheostomy management through design, implementation and prospective audit of a care bundle: how we do it. Clin Otolaryngol 2008;33(5):488–91.
29. Boesch RP, Myers C, Garrett T, et al. Prevention of tracheostomy-related pressure ulcers in children. Pediatrics 2012;129(3):e792–7.
30. Visscher M, King A, Nie AM, et al. A quality-improvement collaborative project to reduce pressure ulcers in PICUs. Pediatrics 2013;131(6):e1950 LP–1960.
31. McEvoy TP, Seim NB, Aljasser A, et al. Prevention of post-operative pediatric tracheotomy wounds: a multidisciplinary team approach. Int J Pediatr Otorhinolaryngol 2017;97:235–9.
32. Helmiö P, Blomgren K, Takala A, et al. Towards better patient safety: WHO surgical safety checklist in otorhinolaryngology. Clin Otolaryngol 2011;36(3):242–7.
33. Soler ZM, Poetker DA, Rudmik L, et al. Multi-institutional evaluation of a sinus surgery checklist. Laryngoscope 2012;122(10):2132–6.

Multidisciplinary Tracheostomy Care

How Collaboratives Drive Quality Improvement

Joshua R. Bedwell, MD, MS[a],
Vinciya Pandian, PhD, MBA, MSN, RN, ACNP-BC[b],
David W. Roberson, MD, MBA, FRCS[c],
Brendan A. McGrath, MBChB, MRCP, FRCA, DICM, EDIC, PGCertMedEd, AHEA,
FFICM, PhD[d], Tanis S. Cameron, MA-SLP (C) CCC-SLP[e],
Michael J. Brenner, MD[f],*

KEYWORDS

- Tracheostomy • Tracheotomy • Quality improvement • Collaborative
- Patient safety

KEY POINTS

- Quality-improvement collaboratives are a powerful mechanism for rapid dissemination and implementation of best practices in patient care to prevent patient harm.
- The Global Tracheostomy Collaborative (GTC) is a quality-improvement collaborative in which member hospitals commit to taking concrete steps to improve the care of tracheostomy patients and track outcomes using a prospective database.
- The 5 key drivers of the GTC are multidisciplinary synchronous ward rounds, standardization of care protocols, appropriate interdisciplinary education, patient and family involvement, and the use of data to drive improvement.

Disclosures: Dr V. Pandian is a consultant for Medtronic and has received a research grant from Smiths Medical. None of the other authors have any commercial or financial disclosures.
[a] Baylor College of Medicine, Texas Children's Hospital, 6701 Fannin Street, Suite 650, Houston, TX 77030, USA; [b] Johns Hopkins School of Nursing, 525 North Wolfe Street, Room 442, Baltimore, MD 21205, USA; [c] Global Tracheostomy Collaborative, 165 Russett Road, West Roxbury, MA 03122, USA; [d] Acute Intensive Care Unit, Wythenshawe Hospital, Manchester University Hospital NHS Foundation Trust, Southmoor Road, Wythenshawe, Manchester, M23 9LT, UK; [e] Austin Health, 3rd Floor Lance Townsend Building, PO Box 5555, Heidelberg, Victoria 3084, Australia; [f] Department of Otolaryngology–Head and Neck Surgery, University of Michigan School of Medicine, 1500 East Medical Center Drive SPC 5312, 1904 Taubman Center, Ann Arbor, MI 48109-5312, USA
* Corresponding author.
E-mail address: mbren@med.umich.edu

Otolaryngol Clin N Am 52 (2019) 135–147
https://doi.org/10.1016/j.otc.2018.08.006
0030-6665/19/© 2018 Elsevier Inc. All rights reserved.

INTRODUCTION

In the United States, greater than 100,000 tracheostomies are performed annually; about 4000 of these are performed in children.[1–3] Extrapolation of survey data on adverse events suggests an annual incidence of approximately 1000 catastrophic tracheostomy-related complications and approximately 500 tracheotomy-related deaths (not all preventable) in the United States.[4] The reported national overall complication rate associated with tracheotomy is 3.2%; but there is marked underreporting of complications, such as emergency tracheostomy tube obstruction or accidental decannulation. Tragically, many catastrophic events and deaths are preventable.[4]

Hospitals in Australia, the United Kingdom, and the United States have demonstrated impressive reductions in untoward outcomes in tracheostomy patients, with an up to 90% decrease in inpatient critical events.[5] Despite very different health care environments and care delivery systems, 5 key elements were present in each successful program: multidisciplinary synchronous ward rounds, standardization of care protocols, appropriate staff training and allocation, patient and family involvement, and use of data to drive improvement.[5–7] Although early experience showing dramatic improvement was first published more than a decade ago, widespread adoption of these practices has not been universal. This finding is not surprising, as some of the practices (eg, multidisciplinary synchronous ward rounds and joint decision-making) represent cultural shifts and, thus, pose significant practical challenges.

One strategy used to accelerate the spread of proven improvement strategies is the quality-improvement collaborative (QIC). First introduced by the Institute for Healthcare Improvement, QICs have been used to drive improvement for many different medical conditions. These endeavors range in size from a set of geographically colocated hospitals within one state to international projects.[8] In a QIC, member hospitals commit to appointing champions and taking specific, concrete steps to accelerate their progress toward the desired state. Participating sites use data to track both the consistency of process changes and the effect on the desired outcomes.[8]

TIMELINE OF THE GLOBAL TRACHEOSTOMY COLLABORATIVE

In 2012, a group of 21 tracheostomy and quality-improvement experts met in Glasgow, Scotland to review the current state of tracheostomy care worldwide. At this initial meeting, the founding members decided to form the Global Tracheostomy Collaborative (GTC), which is now incorporated as a nonprofit corporation in the United States. After the development of a defined improvement strategy and creation of an international, privacy-law-compliant database, the GTC began holding kickoff meetings and enrolling hospital members in 2014.

As of January 2018, the GTC has 45 member hospitals around the world, more than 2000 health care professional members, more than 150 patient and family members, and almost 4000 admissions in its database. The GTC has cohosted 3 International Tracheostomy Symposia, hosts tracheostomy education webinars 8 times annually, and issues biannual data reports. These data allow hospitals to track their progress and to compare their outcomes with other GTC hospitals. Early data have demonstrated significant, meaningful reductions in serious adverse events coupled with improvements in surrogates for the quality and effectiveness of care, such as length of stay within 12 months.[9]

To understand how participation in the collaborative leads to these improvements, it is necessary to understand practical application of the 5 key drivers of tracheostomy care. Each of the 5 subsequent sections focuses on one driver, considering it in the context of the larger initiative. Specific case examples demonstrate implementation of the collaborative across a range of geographies and health care systems. The growing body of data reveal how effective implementation leads to measurable improvements in tracheostomy care across diverse health care systems.[5,6,9,10] This report illustrates how institutions that implemented the key drivers of tracheostomy care improved outcomes within their own institutions and beyond.

COORDINATED MULTIDISCIPLINARY CARE TEAMS: A PERSPECTIVE FROM AUSTIN HEALTH, AUSTRALIA

Austin Health is an academic tertiary health service serving 1.2 million people in Melbourne, Australia. The multidisciplinary Tracheostomy Review and Management Service (TRAMS) was established in 2001 in response to 2 deaths of inpatient tracheostomy patients. TRAMS is a consultative service of tracheostomy specialists, including speech-language pathologists, specialist physiotherapists and intensivists, nurse consultants, and physiotherapists. TRAMS coordinates twice-weekly ward rounds, implements multidisciplinary policy and procedures, and provides education across 3 separate hospital sites, as well as educating within the community. The TRAMS service demonstrated a significant increase in safety and quality-of-life outcomes along with substantial cost savings.[6] The TRAMS team also reported improvements in patient-centered metrics, such as a decrease in time to the first vocalization, shorter time to successful decannulation, and reduction in overall length of stay.[6]

Despite its impressive footprint on tracheostomy care in Australia and globally, TRAMS has a surprisingly small salaried workforce, operating with 2.6 full-time-equivalent staff. Most TRAMS' staff are part-time and also work within other related services. Patients at Austin Health are placed in specialty wards based on their primary diagnosis, regardless of how frequently the specialty ward cares for tracheostomy patients. Therefore, the expertise of the TRAMS team travels to the patients. For instance, liver transplant patients with tracheostomy are placed in the liver transplant ward, where TRAMS provides onsite consultation.

A unique feature of TRAMS at Austin Health is continuity of care. The same clinicians who manage patients in the inpatient setting during an acute admission follow long-term tracheostomy patients into the community. A review of 40 community-based tracheostomy patients in 2012 to 2013 revealed high long-term survival rates with no deaths directly attributed to tracheostomy-related complications.[11] Numerous tracheostomy teams now exist in Australasia based on the TRAMS model, with the body of literature on the effectiveness of such teams growing rapidly.[5,12–15]

At Austin Health, an interdepartmental tracheostomy forum is held twice yearly, whereby all heads of departments and senior staff from relevant disciplines meet to review adverse events, discuss challenging cases, update equipment, and provide cross-discipline education. The TRAMS at Austin Health collaborates with the GTC Patient and Family Committee to Offer Tracheostomy forums twice a year. Up to 75 tracheostomy patients, their families, and professionals meet to share stories, receive awards, and hear presentations on tracheostomy topics. TRAMS patients contribute to the GTC Patient & Family Newsletter and participate in the GTC webinars.

The experience of TRAMS and numerous other GTC member sites suggest that having a physician, a nurse, a respiratory therapist, and a speech-language pathologist as the basic composition of the team in a longitudinal care delivery model leads to improved outcomes.[5–7] The dissemination of Austin Health's practices to other centers in Australasia demonstrates how impact reaches well beyond the confines of the member hospital.

INSTITUTION-WIDE TRACHEOSTOMY PROTOCOLS: AN EXAMPLE FROM THE JOHNS HOPKINS' EXPERIENCE

The Johns Hopkins Hospital has championed the development of several institution-wide tracheostomy protocols to improve patient safety and clinical outcomes. One particularly impactful protocol was the Standardized Tracheostomy Capping and Decannulation Protocol. As with the Austin Health TRAMS initiative, this protocol was developed in response to a root-cause analysis of a significant untoward outcome.[16] The multifaceted protocol not only embraces standardization but also embodies a multidisciplinary team culture in successfully weaning patients from a tracheostomy.

The Development Process

The development of the protocol required the formation of a task force comprising experts from several pertinent disciplines, physicians, nursing, respiratory therapy, and speech-language pathology, as well as the hospital risk manager. Physicians with expertise in otolaryngology, pulmonology, trauma surgery, and anesthesia collaborated. The multidisciplinary task force was led by a tracheostomy nurse practitioner and met bimonthly to create components of the protocol (**Fig. 1**). The team of experts debated and edited each component until consensus was reached. The protocol was then reviewed and revised by the nursing standards of care, medical care evaluation, and medical board administrative committees.

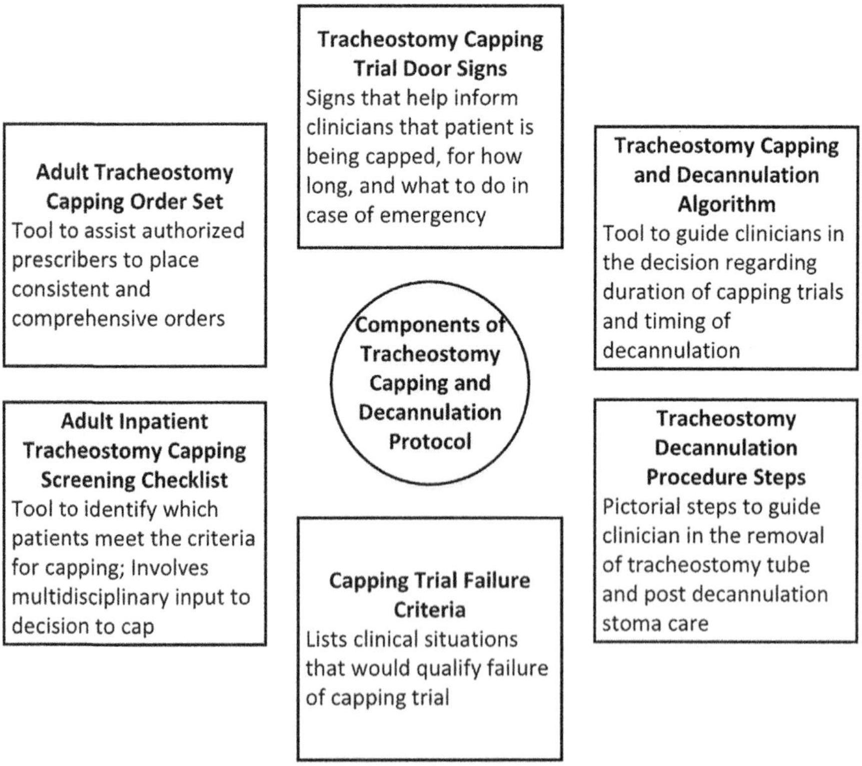

Tracheostomy Capping Trial Door Signs
Signs that help inform clinicians that patient is being capped, for how long, and what to do in case of emergency

Adult Tracheostomy Capping Order Set
Tool to assist authorized prescribers to place consistent and comprehensive orders

Tracheostomy Capping and Decannulation Algorithm
Tool to guide clinicians in the decision regarding duration of capping trials and timing of decannulation

Components of Tracheostomy Capping and Decannulation Protocol

Adult Inpatient Tracheostomy Capping Screening Checklist
Tool to identify which patients meet the criteria for capping; Involves multidisciplinary input to decision to cap

Capping Trial Failure Criteria
Lists clinical situations that would qualify failure of capping trial

Tracheostomy Decannulation Procedure Steps
Pictorial steps to guide clinician in the removal of tracheostomy tube and post decannulation stoma care

Fig. 1. Standardized decannulation protocol components.

Building Awareness

Laying the groundwork for the protocol required attention to education and cultural factors. The process of building awareness about the protocol, creating a sense of urgency around the change, and obtaining buy-in from stakeholders caring for patients throughout the hospital was time consuming. Consistent with many reports from change programs, experienced clinicians were often resistant to change. Certain surgeons did not want to change their approach because of fear of loss of control, whereas some respiratory therapists and nurses were reluctant to provide the extra monitoring or documentation. The multidisciplinary task force met with those resisting change in person or in groups to educate members of the team about the importance of a standardized approach.

Implementation of the Protocol

Implementation of the protocol occurred in 2 phases (**Fig. 2**). In the first phase, the protocol was implemented for a 6-month period in 4 medical/surgical wards after intensive education was provided. Just-in-time education was also provided by the tracheostomy nurse practitioner to strengthen the knowledge about the tracheostomy capping and decannulation protocol once an eligible patient was identified. Based on feedback from the first phase, the protocol was further refined. It was then

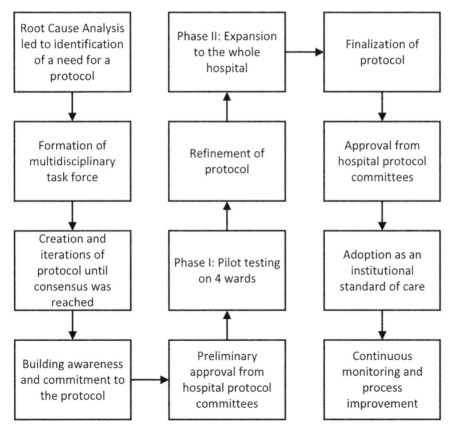

Fig. 2. Development/implementation process for a standardized tracheostomy protocol.

implemented throughout the hospital for the next 6 months to ensure generalizability to other specialty wards and units. On successful implementation throughout the hospital, the protocol was once again reviewed by the stakeholders before adoption as an institutional policy. Experiences of protocol implementation may vary from one institution to another, and member sites can learn from the successes and challenges of those who have put similar protocols into place.

Quality Assurance and Promoting Adherence to Protocol

Adherence to the protocol after the initial implementation phase by all specialties and disciplines is closely monitored by the multidisciplinary tracheostomy team. Adherence to the protocol is reviewed on a weekly basis during weekly tracheostomy rounds. In addition, spot checks are done by the speech-language pathologists and the tracheostomy nurse practitioner. The multidisciplinary tracheostomy team assists the clinicians in the wards with the identification of variations, modification of nursing/rehabilitative activities, and alteration of resource allocation to ensure successful implementation of the protocol.

Multidisciplinary tracheostomy teams can facilitate the development and implementation of standardized protocols, which in turn enable provision of consistent patient care.[17] The tracheostomy protocol created at the Johns Hopkins Hospital is being piloted in several other institutions, including the University of Michigan.

COORDINATED INTERDISCIPLINARY EDUCATION: TEXAS CHILDREN'S HOSPITAL

Children with tracheostomies are a complex and vulnerable population.[4,18] At Texas Children's Hospital (TCH), a multidisciplinary team was developed to evaluate the current state of tracheostomy care, identify targets for improvement, and implement tracheostomy-related initiatives. Here the authors highlight the educational initiatives arising from those efforts.

Nursing Education

Previous studies have described serious deficits in knowledge and comfort with tracheostomy care among health care providers.[19–22] At TCH, a tracheostomy education program consisting of lectures, simulation, and shadowing tracheostomy team rounds was developed by a team of otolaryngology faculty and advanced practice providers. The course resulted in significant improvements in self-efficacy and objective tracheostomy knowledge scores among participating staff (**Figs. 3** and **4**).

Standardized Parent/Caregiver Curriculum

In order to reduce variation in caregiver education from unit to unit before discharge, a workgroup was created to standardize the tracheostomy curriculum. Stakeholders included numerous medical subspecialties (otolaryngology, pulmonology, critical care), nursing representatives from all inpatient wards, speech-language pathology, respiratory therapy, social work, case management, and families and caregivers. The group surveyed all tracheostomy educational materials and then worked together to develop a caregiver handbook.

The resulting handbook is a comprehensive resource for parents, used from presurgery discussions through discharge and outpatient care. Including all stakeholders at the outset was key in obtaining buy-in from units accustomed to their own policies and procedures. Families ensured the handbook covered high-yield topics and explained concepts and procedures in understandable language.

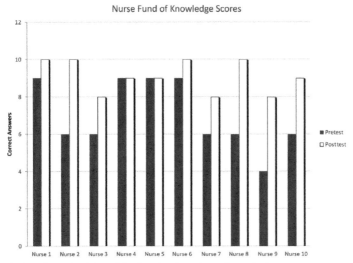

Fig. 3. Pretest and posttest for objective tracheostomy knowledge.

Simulation in Parent/Caregiver Education

Although simulation is pervasive in medical education, reports of its use in educating patients and caregivers are limited.[23,24] At TCH, a simulation-based educational program (the Parent Emergency Preparedness for Tracheostomy Assisted Living and Care program) was created based on feedback from recently discharged families.[25] Before discharge, all caregivers of new tracheostomy patients must complete the 4-hour course, which includes 4 scenarios: blocked tracheostomy tube, dislodged tube, water in the ventilator tubing, and cardiac arrest. Debriefing is performed with

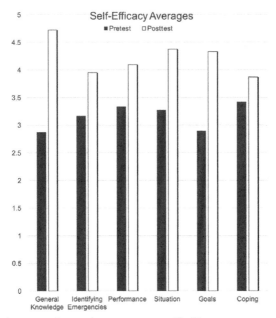

Fig. 4. Pretest and posttest for tracheostomy care self-efficacy.

trained simulation educators, and learners have the ability to repeat scenarios until competency is obtained. Preliminary data support the salutary effects of simulation on caregiver knowledge and confidence. Other institutions are developing simulation-based tracheostomy programs; the GTC provides a venue for dialogue among member sites and promotes the rapid sharing of ideas and materials related to developing a comprehensive and effective tracheostomy curriculum.

PATIENT- AND FAMILY CENTERED CARE: UNIVERSITY OF MICHIGAN, UNITED KINGDOM, AND BEYOND

The patient advocacy credo, *nothing about us without us*, emphasizes the desire of patients and their caregivers to participate in decision-making. High-quality care is fostered by seeking patient perspectives, inviting feedback, and developing patient-centered performance measures.[26] As the Agency for Healthcare Research and Quality notes, patient engagement promotes measurable improvements in safety and quality.[27] Patients and caregivers are an integral part of the GTC, and the collaborative prioritizes clinical outcomes based on such input.

Patients and families emphasize that excellent tracheostomy care focuses on quality of life, rather than solely avoidance of complications. Multidisciplinary teams can promote patient-centered care outcomes, such as restoring speech. Timely speech rehabilitation after tracheostomy may seem less pressing than other medical interventions, but aphonic patients are vulnerable and in significant psychological distress. Impaired speech and communication after tracheostomy can lead to social withdrawal and compromised emotional well-being.[28,29] Patients who cannot speak are unable to call for help during a medical emergency. A team-based approach led to improved use of one-way speaking valves, which was associated with decreased adverse events, decreased length of stay, and shorter duration of cannulation.[30]

Patients and their families also can experience frustration, particularly in areas such as impaired communication with the care team or difficulty in securing necessary medical supplies. At the University of Michigan, patients and caregivers are integrated into a tracheostomy trail, a detailed framework for orchestrating care from before tracheostomy through discharge, with iterative assessment of patient needs and training. Involving patients in these efforts along with physicians in training has a lasting impact on culture and quality-improvement efforts.[31]

Social media platforms incorporating patients and family also provide improvement opportunities. One survey of patients and families with tracheostomy found that only half of respondents had the opportunity to meet with a patient with a tracheostomy before surgery or felt prepared to handle tracheostomy care at the time of discharge.[32] Patients and families noted difficulty in securing products and services relating to the tracheostomy care. Such difficulties are more than inconveniences, as they risk the loss of life in the event of tracheostomy occlusion or malfunction.[4] The collaborative provides a forum for patients to share experiences among themselves and with the medical community.

The National Tracheostomy Safety Project (NSTP) in the United Kingdom affords a perspective on the impressive reach of social media–based strategies. This NTSP developed a marketing campaign to target key staff groups with easily digestible tracheostomy safety resources. The strategy was built around understanding the audience (what they wanted and how they wanted to consume resources), developing high-quality content to convey key messages, and then targeting frontline staff through a mixture of native and promoted social media activity. This approach resulted in far more interaction than publishing an article in a journal. For example, as of this writing, the "Multidisciplinary Emergency Tracheostomy Guidelines" article that underpinned this project has been cited in the medical literature 89 times since publication in September 2012.[33] This figure is dwarfed by responses from the 2018 social media project, totaling 629,270 social media impressions of the newly created video and infographic resources. Where user profile data were available, most impressions were viewed by bedside health care staff (nurses, respiratory therapists, speech-language pathologists), with around two-thirds of impressions shared between peers, demonstrating significant engagement and social mobilization around the content and these themes. Patients and their families/caregivers also engaged through established and personal social media groups, one of the highlights of working in this multidisciplinary partnership. Involving family members in education and decision-making at every step possible is empowering and can help clinicians meet patient and family expectations while ensuring mastery of key competencies.

DATA COLLECTION AND TRACKING OUTCOMES: MULTIHOSPITAL INITIATIVES IN THE UNITED KINGDOM

Accurate and meaningful data are essential in determining the impact of quality-improvement interventions. The ideal tracheostomy-related data collection tools will track patient-level metrics that can inform medical institutions about progress and performance at ward level (reductions in harm or provision of essential equipment), at a system level (reductions in length of stay or readmission rates), or metrics that reflect quality of care (early vocalization or oral intake). As alluded to in the prior section, patients and their families often describe very different performance metrics to those that would seem important to health care providers.[34]

The GTC Database Committee created a robust, Health Insurance Portability and Accountability Act (HIPAA)–compliant database for prospectively following tracheostomy outcomes. The database was created by expert volunteers from 9 disciplines and has been in use for more than 5 years and now has about 4000 entries (**Fig. 5**). Biannual reports are provided to member institutions with their own data and aggregate data of all sites.

An important element of data collection is establishing who collects the data, where, and when. In the United Kingdom, the GTC has worked with more than 25 hospitals in establishing the most effective methods of data collection. Member institutions have attempted a variety of methods, from dedicated data clerks to senior medical staff. Although it may only take a few minutes to physically enter the data, identifying and tracking patients through their hospital stay can be a challenge for busy clinical teams.[10] A degree of topic-specific medical knowledge is often required for meaningful data collection. The relative importance of a specific metric must be balanced against the accuracy and ease of its collection.

In a detailed analysis of the data collection of 4 UK sites participating in the GTC, data quality was found to be high. A total of 918 of 934 (98.3%) of new cases had the basic mandatory data set completed.[9] The UK group also met and worked through a consensus exercise to agree on the priority and order in which interventions would be attempted and which metrics would be collected to track their progress. As a result, member institutions reported a degree of ownership and buy-in to the project and did not think that they were collecting irrelevant data or undertaking interventions that were not considered useful at their site.[34]

Analyses of the GTC projects in the National Health System of the United Kingdom have demonstrated improvements across domains, including safer care, reduced length of stay, and shorter times to vocalization and established oral intake following

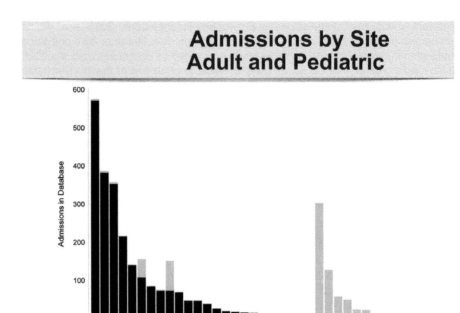

Fig. 5. GTC database entries categorized by adult versus pediatric patients. (*Courtesy of* Global Tracheostomy Collaborative, http://globaltrach.org; with permission.)

tracheostomy. The ability to benchmark these metrics over time and to compare them with other similar sites will be a welcome addition, making comparisons increasingly valid and meaningful as the database grows. Future targets are likely to arise from the current 3-year Improving Tracheostomy Care project in the United Kingdom, where a target of 1200 health care staff, patients, and their families will be asked about the difficulties in providing and receiving safe, high-quality care. As an example of how improvement collaboratives like the GTC can be responsive to the needs of participating sites and their patients, future metrics can be defined and refined through an active social media community, involving both care providers and patients themselves.

SYNTHESIS AND SUMMARY

The preceding examples of institutions implementing the key drivers of the GTC exemplify change agents who have not only made an impact within their institution but also disseminated these practices to peer institutions.

Collaboratives are learning communities that drive positive change through effective communication, dissemination, and implementation of proven strategies. In the case of the GTC, this learning occurs through sharing of ideas between institutions via discussion boards, live webinars, and the International Tracheostomy Symposia. Standardized hospital protocols, policies, and procedures are easily shared online with other member hospitals. Patients and caregivers access these same platforms to share their perspectives with each other and the medical professionals involved in their care. The direct, ongoing interaction afforded by the GTC ensures a continued focus on patient-centered outcomes.[32,35]

Communicating data is critical. The GTC database has been refined to reflect the needs of its users, affording institutions an easy way to track their own outcomes;

pooling data can help in identifying trends that may not be apparent on a small scale. Members are able to easily recognize targets for improvement when they can see how their own outcomes are situated in the context of other member hospitals. Such benchmarking may also prove useful when requesting additional funding or resources for a tracheostomy program. Sharing best practices in tracheostomy will likely increasingly involve engaging with social media. This future is already becoming reality with initiatives emerging in the United Kingdom.

In summary, adopting the 5 key drivers of the GTC has proven highly effective for a wide range of international institutions who are improving the care of patients with tracheostomies. These drivers serve as a framework for assessing the current quality of care and for designing targeted interventions. A universal theme in all examples is the importance of the multidisciplinary team. Although the benefits of coordinated multidisciplinary tracheostomy teams appeared in the literature before the formation of the GTC,[12] these reports did not result in broad adoption. The creation and growth of the QIC created a community of like-minded members, who now have a platform for sharing and a record of measurable, lasting improvements in outcomes being tracked on a large-scale basis.

REFERENCES

1. Agency for Healthcare Research and Quality. Statistics on hospital stays. 2014. Available at: http://hcupnet.ahrq.gov/HCUPnet.jsp?Id=6F3B8F3A0A992F7D&. Accessed October 6, 2014.
2. Cheung NH, Napolitano LM. Tracheostomy: epidemiology, indications, timing, technique, and outcomes. Respir Care 2014;59(6):895–915 [discussion: 916–9].
3. Shah RK, Lander L, Berry JG, et al. Tracheotomy outcomes and complications: a national perspective. Laryngoscope 2012;122(1):25–9.
4. Das P, Zhu H, Shah RK, et al. Tracheotomy-related catastrophic events: results of a national survey. Laryngoscope 2012;122(1):30–7.
5. Cetto R, Arora A, Hettige R, et al. Improving tracheostomy care: a prospective study of the multidisciplinary approach. Clin Otolaryngol 2011;36(5):482–8.
6. Cameron TS, McKinstry A, Burt SK, et al. Outcomes of patients with spinal cord injury before and after introduction of an interdisciplinary tracheostomy team. Crit Care Resusc 2009;11(1):14–9.
7. Pandian V, Miller CR, Mirski MA, et al. Multidisciplinary team approach in the management of tracheostomy patients. Otolaryngol Head Neck Surg 2012; 147(4):684–91.
8. The breakthrough series: IHI's collaborative model for achieving breakthrough improvement. IHI innovation series white paper. Boston: Institute for Healthcare Improvement; 2003.
9. McGrath BA, Lynch J, Bonvento B, et al. Evaluating the quality improvement impact of the Global Tracheostomy Collaborative in four diverse NHS hospitals. BMJ Qual Improv Rep 2017;6(1) [pii:bmjqir.u220636.w7996].
10. Lavin J, Shah R, Greenlick H, et al. The global tracheostomy collaborative: one institution's experience with a new quality improvement initiative. Int J Pediatr Otorhinolaryngol 2016;80:106–8.
11. Lim MCT, McMurray K, Chao C, et al. Outcomes of patients living with a tracheostomy in the community. 2nd International Tracheostomy Symposium. Melbourne, Australia, October 8, 2014.

12. Garrubba M, Turner T, Grieveson C. Multidisciplinary care for tracheostomy patients: a systematic review. Crit Care 2009;13(6):R177.
13. Speed L, Harding KE. Tracheostomy teams reduce total tracheostomy time and increase speaking valve use: a systematic review and meta-analysis. J Crit Care 2013;28(2):216.e1-10.
14. Yaneza MM, James HP, Davies P, et al. Changing indications for paediatric tracheostomy and the role of a multidisciplinary tracheostomy clinic. J Laryngol Otol 2015;129(9):882–6.
15. Abode KA, Drake AF, Zdanski CJ, et al. A multidisciplinary children's airway center: impact on the care of patients with tracheostomy. Pediatrics 2016;137(2): e20150455.
16. Pandian V, Miller CR, Schiavi AJ, et al. Utilization of a standardized tracheostomy capping and decannulation protocol to improve patient safety. Laryngoscope 2014;124(8):1794–800.
17. Mitchell R, Parker V, Giles M. An interprofessional team approach to tracheostomy care: a mixed-method investigation into the mechanisms explaining tracheostomy team effectiveness. Int J Nurs Stud 2013;50(4):536–42.
18. Mahida JB, Asti L, Boss EF, et al. Tracheostomy placement in children younger than 2 years: 30-day outcomes using the national surgical quality improvement program pediatric. JAMA Otolaryngol Head Neck Surg 2016;142(3):241–6.
19. Dorton LH, Lintzenich CR, Evans AK. Simulation model for tracheotomy education for primary health-care providers. Ann Otol Rhinol Laryngol 2014;123(1): 11–8.
20. Yelverton JC, Nguyen JH, Wan W, et al. Effectiveness of a standardized education process for tracheostomy care. Laryngoscope 2015;125(2):342–7.
21. McGrath B, Wilkinson K, Shah RK. Notes from a small island: lessons from the UK NCEPOD tracheotomy report. Otolaryngol Head Neck Surg 2015;153(2):167–9.
22. Agarwal A, Marks N, Wessel V, et al. Improving knowledge, technical skills, and confidence among pediatric health care providers in the management of chronic tracheostomy using a simulation model. Pediatr Pulmonol 2016;51(7):696–704.
23. Coleman EA. Extending simulation learning experiences to patients with chronic health conditions. JAMA 2014;311(3):243–4.
24. Sigalet E, Cheng A, Donnon T, et al. A simulation-based intervention teaching seizure management to caregivers: a randomized controlled pilot study. Paediatr Child Health 2014;19(7):373–8.
25. Arnold J, Diaz MC. Simulation training for primary caregivers in the neonatal intensive care unit. Semin Perinatol 2016;40(7):466–72.
26. Ward E, Pandian V, Brenner MJ. The primacy of patient-centered outcomes in tracheostomy care. Patient 2018;11(2):143–5.
27. Agency for Healthcare Research and Quality. Guide to patient and family engagement in hospital quality and safety. 2013. Available at: http://www.ahrq. gov/professionals/systems/hospital/engagingfamilies/guide.html. Accessed March 15, 2018.
28. Nakarada-Kordic I, Patterson N, Wrapson J, et al. A systematic review of patient and caregiver experiences with a tracheostomy. Patient 2018;11(2):175–91.
29. Pritchett CV, Foster Rietz M, Ray A, et al. Inpatient nursing and parental comfort in managing pediatric tracheostomy care and emergencies. JAMA Otolaryngol Head Neck Surg 2016;142(2):132–7.
30. Cameron M, Corner A, Diba A, et al. Development of a tracheostomy scoring system to guide airway management after major head and neck surgery. Int J Oral Maxillofac Surg 2009;38(8):846–9.

31. Morrison RJ, Bowe SN, Brenner MJ. Teaching quality improvement and patient safety in residency education: strategies for meaningful resident quality and safety initiatives. JAMA Otolaryngol Head Neck Surg 2017;143(11):1069–70.
32. McCormick ME, Ward E, Roberson DW, et al. Life after tracheostomy: patient and family perspectives on teaching, transitions, and multidisciplinary teams. Otolaryngol Head Neck Surg 2015;153(6):914–20.
33. McGrath BA, Bates L, Atkinson D, et al. Multidisciplinary guidelines for the management of tracheostomy and laryngectomy airway emergencies. Anaesthesia 2012;67(9):1025–41.
34. McGrath BL J, Coe B, Wallace S, et al. Improving tracheostomy care: collaborative national consensus and prioritisation of quality improvements in the United Kingdom. Med Res Arch 2018;6(1):1–10.
35. Wilkinson KA, Martin IC, Freeth H, et al. NCEPOD: on the right Trach? 2014. Available at: www.ncepod.org.uk/2014tc.htm. Accessed March 15, 2018.

Button Battery Safety
Industry and Academic Partnerships to Drive Change

Kris R. Jatana, MD[a,b,]*, Silas Chao, BS[c], Ian N. Jacobs, MD[d,e],
Toby Litovitz, MD[f]

KEYWORDS

- Button battery • Disc battery • Coin cell battery • Injury prevention • Esophageal
- Foreign body

KEY POINTS

- The enormous number of button batteries (BB) in circulation continues to grow, and BB injuries in children continue to be a source of morbidity and mortality.
- When lodged in the body, BB can cause serious injury in a matter of hours by creating a highly alkaline caustic injury with local tissue pH 10 to 13.
- Early detection and prompt removal are critical to achieving best outcomes.
- Based on recent research, novel mitigation strategies, including pre-removal honey or Carafate, to decrease the rate of initial injury and post-removal esophageal pH neutralization with 0.25% acetic acid irrigation reduces the likelihood of progressive liquefactive tissue necrosis.
- Organized national collaborative efforts with all stakeholders involved with the BB problem continues to help identify and drive interventions to help reduce injury risk to children.

Disclosure Statement: K.R. Jatana serves as a general product safety medical consultant for Intertek Inc. K.R. Jatana has a patent pending coin/battery metal detector device under development, which is discussed in this article. K.R. Jatana receives royalties for a patented, commercially available medical device, not related to nor discussed in this article from Marpac Inc. Both K.R. Jatana and I.N. Jacobs serve in leadership positions on the National Button Battery Task Force, supported by and affiliated with the American Academy of Pediatrics and American Broncho-Esophagological Association. The authors have no other potential funding, financial relationships, or conflicts of interest to disclose.
[a] Department of Pediatric Otolaryngology, Nationwide Children's Hospital, 555 South 18th Street, Suite 2A, Columbus, OH 43205, USA; [b] Department of Otolaryngology–Head and Neck Surgery, Wexner Medical Center at Ohio State University, 915 Olentangy River Road, Columbus, OH 43212, USA; [c] Northeast Ohio Medical University, 4209 State Route 44, P.O. Box 95, Rootstown, OH 44272, USA; [d] Division of Pediatric Otolaryngology, Children's Hospital of Philadelphia, 3401 Civic Center Boulevard, Philadelphia, PA 19104, USA; [e] Department of Otorhinolaryngology–Head and Neck Surgery, Perelman School of Medicine, University of Pennsylvania, 3400 Civic Center Boulevard, Philadelphia, PA 19104, USA; [f] National Capital Poison Center, 3201 New Mexico Avenue Northwest #310, Washington, DC 20016, USA
* Corresponding author. Department of Pediatric Otolaryngology, Nationwide Children's Hospital, 555 South 18th Street, Suite 2A, Columbus, OH 43205.
E-mail address: Kris.Jatana@nationwidechildrens.org

Otolaryngol Clin N Am 52 (2019) 149–161
https://doi.org/10.1016/j.otc.2018.08.009
0030-6665/19/© 2018 Elsevier Inc. All rights reserved.

HISTORICAL PERSPECTIVE

Button batteries (BB) were first produced in volume in the late 1950s. In 1945, Ruben and Mallory, which would later become Duracell, invented the zinc-mercuric oxide alkaline button-type cell.[1] The development of miniaturized batteries and electronics advanced together as Eveready introduced the first BB for hearing aids in 1955 and later introduced the first commercial watch BB in 1957.[2] BB technology continued to improve as Eveready produced the first silver oxide system of BB in 1960 for hearing aids.[2] The silver oxide BB enabled more compact design in electronic devices such as watches.[3,4] However, rising silver prices during 1979 led to an increase in the price of silver oxide batteries.[4] This led to the development and increased production of alkaline manganese BB and lithium BB.[4] Today, alkaline manganese BB are still seen commonly in some wristwatches, clocks, and musical greeting cards. Lithium chemistry was actually used in the US space program in the 1950s.[4] Today, lithium BBs are popular, as they have 3 V, a long shelf life, and the largest capacitance in relation to their size.[4,5] The chemistry within lithium batteries varies with manganese dioxide, fluorographite, copper oxide, thionyl chloride, and sulfur dioxide. The CR2032 is the most commonly used lithium coin cell today, and it has a high potential risk of serious injury after ingestion.[6–9] The "CR" is the chemical identification for lithium/manganese dioxide and the "2032" defines a diameter of 20 mm, a thickness of 3.2 mm.[5]

The use of mercury in consumer batteries has declined sharply in the United States. Currently, only small amounts of mercury are incorporated in BBs to inhibit internal gas formation, which is suspected to cause bulging and potentially result in leakage of battery contents.[10,11] The toxicity of mercury to the environment was recognized nationally and eventually led to the passage of the *Mercury-Containing and Rechargeable Battery Management Act* in 1996, which phased-out mercuric oxide batteries.[12,13] In addition to the environmental hazard, it is known that mercury poisoning can cause systemic injuries, including those to the gastrointestinal tract, central nervous system, and kidneys. Nonetheless, no cases of symptomatic mercury poisoning have been reported following mercury battery ingestion.

The 4 major types of BB chemistry are used today: lithium, zinc air, alkaline, and silver oxide.[10] Although larger diameter, 3 V lithium BBs pose the greatest risk of becoming lodged and causing injury in the esophagus, the risk of smaller diameter, lower-voltage non-lithium BBs cannot be ignored, as they can cause severe injury and complications, just at a slower rate.[14]

IMPACT OF BUTTON BATTERIES ON CHILDREN

Although this is clearly a worldwide problem, more than 3000 BB ingestions are reported annually in the United States.[15] When a child ingests a BB, significant esophageal injury can occur within 2 hours. The resulting alkaline reaction on the mucosal tissue is due to hydrolysis of water generating hydroxide ions at the negative terminal or anode leading to a subsequent rise in pH and liquefactive tissue necrosis.[14,16] The ensuing complications from BB ingestion continue to be a significant cause of morbidity and mortality. In an analysis by the National Battery Ingestion Hotline (NBIH) for battery ingestion in children younger than 6 years old, 61.8% of ingested batteries were obtained directly from the product by the child, 29.8% were loose, sitting out, or discarded, and 8.2% were obtained from battery packaging.[9] In the same analysis, an alarming 12.6% of children younger than 6 years who ingested 20-mm-diameter lithium BBs experienced a major complication, such as a perforation, tracheoesophageal fistula, fistulization into major vessels, esophageal strictures, vocal cord paralysis, or spondylodiscitis.[9] Since 1977, there have been at least 59 reported fatalities from BB ingestion.[17]

PRIOR PROGRESS

The NBIH was created in 1982 to help gather case data, create triage algorithms, and identify methods of reducing this hazard. This hotline is available 24/7 and provides the public as well as health care providers with guidance when a battery-related injury is suspected. Updated statistics are available at www.poison.org/battery.

On March 1, 1983, the US Consumer Product Safety Commission (CPSC) issued a warning on BBs.[18] In February 2010, a statement from the Dry Battery Section of the National Electrical Manufacturers Association (NEMA), highlighted the known serious health consequences to unintentional ingestion of BBs.[19]

In June 2010, informative articles were published in the medical literature from the National Capital Poison Center.[8] The trends of moderate, major, and fatal outcomes are best demonstrated in **Fig. 1**. Between 2003 and 2007, there was a dramatic increase in the number of injuries from BB ingestion. There are several datasets that have been used nationally to track the injuries from BBs.

On March 17, 2011, there was joint presentation by 2 future leading members (Jatana KR and Litovitz T) of the National Button Battery Task Force (BBTF) at the CPSC.[20] As a result, on March 23, 2011, an additional CPSC alert went out to urge members of industry to become more aware of the hazard of BBs to children. In June 2011, the *Button Cell Battery Safety Act* was proposed, but Congress never enacted the bill. That bill would have required the CPSC to enforce consumer product safety standards that require child-resistant battery compartment closures on consumer products containing BBs.[21] The legislation failed to advance past Senate Subcommittee. In-person lobbying efforts with members of Congress in Washington, DC, were carried out by several pediatric otolaryngologists.

In 2012, the Centers for Disease Control and Prevention published a report of injuries from 1995 to 2010 related to BBs, and stated, "Injuries to children caused by batteries have been documented in the medical literature and by poison control centers for decades."[22] Simultaneously in 2012, the National BBTF was formalized

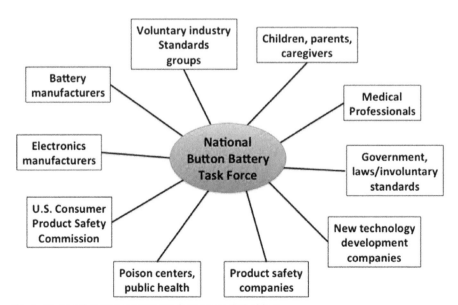

Fig. 1. National Button Battery Task Force Stakeholders.

within the American Academy of Pediatrics (AAP) and the American Broncho-Esophagological Association (ABEA) with a central mission statement:

A collaborative effort of representatives from relevant organizations in industry, medicine, public health, and government to develop, coordinate, and implement strategies to reduce the incidence of button battery injuries in children.

CONTINUED PROGRESS OF NATIONAL BUTTON BATTERY TASK FORCE

Since formalization of the National BBTF in 2012, we have reviewed the BB injury prevention interventions. These specific multipronged efforts have involved collaboration with key stakeholders related to the BB problem (see **Fig. 1**). Over the past several years, the national BBTF has helped influence several notable safety changes. These are summarized in **Table 1** and further discussed later in this article. The reported national ingestion trends, as well as those children having complications, are shown in **Fig. 2**.

CONSUMER AWARENESS

Members of the BBTF have increased the public and medical community awareness of this hazard through organized media efforts (radio, print, online, social media, television), which have had both national and international impact. In 2011, Energizer and other safety-oriented partners launched "The Battery Controlled" public awareness campaign for consumer education of this hazard. In general, consumer education is critical with regard to injury prevention. If consumers, especially parents and childcare providers, are NOT aware of the hazard, they cannot help with primary prevention of the injuries.

EDUCATION OF MEDICAL PROFESSIONALS

The AAP has taken a lead in helping educate pediatric medical professionals, with a focus on emergency and urgent care providers, radiologists, surgeons, gastroenterologists, and anesthesiologists, helping to keep all these medical professionals up to date with the latest management protocols. The most reliable radiographic finding to differentiate a BB from a coin, is to zoom in and observe the double ring/halo sign on the anterior-posterior radiograph (**Fig. 3**). The lateral radiograph alone with slimmer BBs may not consistently have a step-off and appears no different from a coin.[16] Over the years, National BBTF-related presentations, panels, or mini-seminars have been done at the American College of Surgeons, American Broncho-Esophagological Association, American Society of Pediatric Otolaryngology, European Society of Pediatric Otorhinolaryngology, and American Academy of Otolaryngology–Head and Neck Surgery to help educate medical professionals with the latest management strategies when ingestions occur. **Table 2** highlights the latest updates on clinical management considerations for BB ingestions. The latest National Capital Poison Center Battery Guidelines, can be reviewed at: https://www.poison.org/battery/guideline.

PACKAGING CHANGES

Battery manufactures, such as Duracell and Energizer, have improved their packaging to consist of double packaging around the battery.[23] This change requires the use of a scissor for the initial removal of the battery from the packaging, making access to batteries harder for children.[24,25] The battery industry as a whole has also taken

Table 1
Multipronged interventions for injury mitigation

Category	Intervention(s)
Education	Hazard awareness to parents, caregivers, day cares, babysitter class curriculums. Online information on National Button Battery Task Force Web site within www.aap.org and www.healthychildren.org. • Store new button batteries (BBs) in a secured container, out of reach of children. • Thoroughly examine all electronics in the home setting to ensure BBs are contained in a secure compartment, and monitor these products over time to ensure the compartment stays secure. • Properly dispose of or recycle old BBs immediately after removing from a device that contains replaceable BB. Distribution of relevant, updated clinical information to medical professionals. For the latest National Capital Poison Center Battery Guidelines, please visit: https://www.poison.org/battery/guideline.
Warning labels	Improved warnings on BB packaging and products that contain them. Pictogram stickers on negative pole of battery, require consumer removal before use in a device.
Secure battery packaging	Some brands require scissors to cut packaging and access batteries. Some brands incorporate individual compartments for each BB, so all cannot fall out at once.
Product safety standards	Legislation Button Cell Battery Safety Act 2011-*failed.* Mandatory Industry Standard American Society for Testing and Materials (ASTM) F 963–17, Toy Standard Voluntary Industry Standards. American National Standards Institute/Underwriters Laboratories (ANSI/UL) 60065: Standard for Audio, Visual, and Similar Electronic Apparatus–Safety Requirements. ANSI/UL 4200A: Standard for Safety for Products Incorporating Button Cell Batteries of Lithium and Similar Technologies.
Early detection screening methods	Novel coin-BB metal detector screening technology in development, patent pending. Ability for rapid, zero-radiation screening of children with nonspecific symptoms of foreign body ingestion, such as fever, poor mouth intake, cough, difficulty swallowing, sore throat, or wheezing who present to primary care offices, urgent cares, emergency rooms.
Slowing progression of injury	Esophageal tissue pH neutralization pre-removal (honey in home setting; sucralfate/Carafate® or honey in clinical setting).[26] Esophageal tissue pH neutralization irrigation post-removal (0.25% sterile acetic acid).[14]
Protocols to expedite care	Improving communication pathways, sharing of institutional protocols, electronic medical record interventions, current American College of Surgeon's National Surgical Quality Improvement Program Pediatric Process Measure.
Changing BB design	The National BBTF *strongly supports* any development effort to modify the BB design so it *does not cause injury* while in the body.

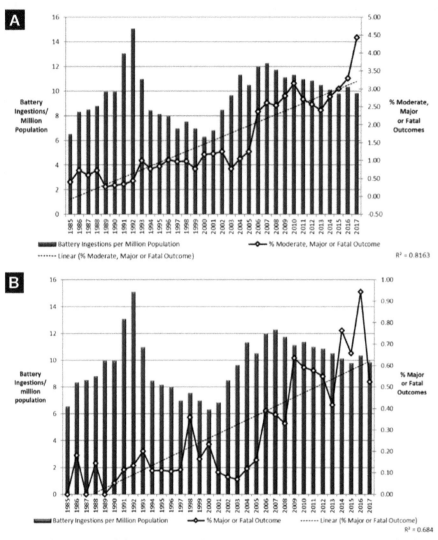

Fig. 2. Updated national data on reported BB ingestions. (*A*) Moderate, major, or fatal outcomes. (*B*) Major or fatal outcomes only.

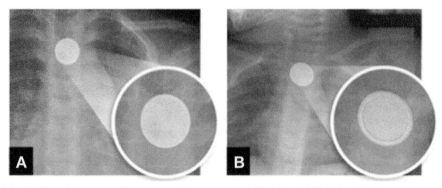

Fig. 3. On radiographs, always zoom in to any metallic object. (*A*) Coin with homogeneous appearance. (*B*) BB with double ring or halo. (*Courtesy of* K.R. Jatana, MD, Columbus, OH.)

Table 2
Clinical considerations for pre-removal, at time of removal in operating room, and post-removal

Pre-removal Early stage ingestions	If no clinical suspicion of delayed diagnosis (<12 hours since ingestion), existing esophageal perforation, mediastinitis, or sepsis, consider these interventions shown to decrease rate of injury[26] • In a home setting, consider honey, 10 mL (2 teaspoons) every 10 min, up to 6 doses, until patient arrives at a hospital. Avoid honey in children <1 year old. • In a clinical setting, consider sucralfate (Carafate®) or honey, 10 mL (2 teaspoons) every 10 min, up to 3 doses, until button battery (BB) can be removed. Avoid honey in children <1 year old. These interventions are NOT a substitute for prompt removal.
Operating room	Surgical emergency, done regardless of NPO (nothing by mouth) status. Rapid sequence induction. Expedite getting to operating room for BB removal. Consider doing direct laryngoscopy and bronchoscopy to evaluate for laryngotracheal airway injury, especially in cases in which negative pole is anterior (step-off anterior). Consider potential complications, such as esophageal perforation, tracheoesophageal fistula, vocal cord paresis or paralysis, and proximity to major vascular structures. If no visible esophageal perforation, endoscopic irrigation of site of injury with 50–150 mL of 0.25% sterile acetic acid, suction simultaneously out.[14]
Post-removal	Consider esophagram before oral intake to rule out perforation. Consider contrast imaging of chest (MRI, computed tomography angiography) if severe injury exists and concern for proximity to major vascular structures (eg, aorta). Monitor for potential complications, such as delayed esophageal perforation, tracheo-esophageal fistula, aorto-esophageal fistula, vocal cord paresis or paralysis, mediastinitis, spondylodiscitis, or esophageal stricture.

significant measures to limit the risk of battery ingestion, such as more clear warnings on packaging, a warning sticker on the battery, or in some cases an engraved warning on the battery surface (**Fig. 4**).

INDUSTRY STANDARDS

BB manufactures have worked with the International Electrotechnical Commission and other standards-setting organizations, such as Underwriters Laboratories (UL) and the American National Standards Institute (ANSI) to ensure secure battery compartments in battery-powered electronics. Specifically, ANSI/UL 60065: Standard

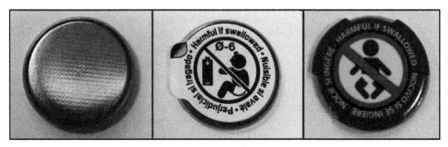

Fig. 4. Warning label stickers on negative pole of some BBs.

for Audio, Video and Similar Electronic Apparatus–Safety Requirements (2014) and ANSI/UL 4200A: Standard for Safety for Products that Incorporate Button or Coin Cell Batteries Using Lithium Technologies (2015) were created for electronic devices that contain lithium BB. These standards require that the BB must be contained in the device and a tool or a minimum of 2 simultaneous independent movements be required to gain access to it. A similar standard is currently being considered for all products containing nonlithium chemistry BBs, given they have also caused serious injuries in children.

On January 25, 2017, the CPSC voted unanimously to approve the revised American Society for Testing and Materials (ASTM) F963-16 as a *mandatory* toy safety standard; this requires that toys designed for use by children younger than 14 years have a warning label on packaging and additional instructions to alert the consumer to the hazard of the BB. This also incorporates new testing requirements for BB 1.5 V and greater: overcharging, repetitive overcharging, single fault charging tests, and short circuit protection tests. This *new mandatory standard* became effective on April 30, 2017.[27]

PRODUCTS AS A SOURCE

Most ingested BBs come from products themselves, and lists of more common electronics are shown in **Tables 3** and **4**. The impact of the new standards has not yet been determined. The challenge is that complete replacement of older products in the household with industry-standard–compliant products takes time.

EARLY DETECTION

The concept of early detection of esophageal BBs, especially in unwitnessed cases in which children may present with nonspecific symptoms, has led to the development of new patent-pending technology at Nationwide Children's and Ohio State, which has not only the ability to detect a coin or BB in the esophagus, but the ability to tell the user a coin versus a BB. Unless acute respiratory distress is present, coins can be observed and removed electively, whereas BBs require emergent removal. **Fig. 5** demonstrates the potential clinical utility of such a device. It has been determined that current handheld metal detectors for security purposes are not sensitive enough for the deeper detection of mid-distal esophageal coins or BBs.[28] It will also pick up unwitnessed ingestions of coins lodged in the esophagus. At this time, commercialization opportunities are being explored for the creation of a reliable pediatric foreign body screening technology.

QUALITY IMPROVEMENT

Expedited care for children with an esophageal BB is critical to optimizing outcomes. The use of Trauma 1 activation has been shown to lead to shorter times to removal when compared with standard emergency room triage.[29] Clinical factors that are predictive for long-term complications have also been investigated. The esophageal location and orientation of the BB negative pole, the anatomic location of the most severe esophageal injuries, the estimated time of impaction, and the characteristics of the specific battery should be used to guide further management and follow-up.[30] Time from radiographic diagnosis to operating room for esophageal BB cases was recently selected as a pilot American College of Surgeon's National Surgical Quality Improvement Program Pediatric Process Measure. These pilot data are currently being collected at participating pediatric centers. This may provide pediatric centers with awareness of where their process stands for emergent BB removal and may be a future opportunity for centers to learn from others.

Table 3
Intended use of ingested button batteries, all types, July 2014 to June 2016

Intended Use	Frequency	Percent	Valid Percent
Alarm	7	0.3	0.4
Book light	14	0.6	0.8
Book: talking/singing	6	0.3	0.3
Calculator	21	0.9	1.2
Candle (flameless, tea)	22	1.0	1.3
Car remote, key fob; keyless entry	11	0.5	0.6
Card: singing/talking	3	0.1	0.2
Clock/timer	10	0.4	0.6
Cochlear implant	4	0.2	0.2
Flashing/musical accessories	8	0.3	0.5
Game/toy	420	18.2	24.1
Hearing aid	580	25.1	33.3
Jewelry: lighted	16	0.7	0.9
Lights	330	14.3	19.0
Finger light	29	1.3	1.7
Flashlight (including toy flashlights, pen lights)	158	6.8	9.1
Keychain light or other	37	1.6	2.1
Laser light, pointer, or pen	70	3.0	4.0
Miscellaneous lights	36	1.6	2.1
Bike light (1); camping light stick (1); fishing pole light (1); glow stick (1); head lamp (2); night light (4); reading light (4)			
Meters/gauges/tools/medical devices	12	0.5	0.7
Dental tool (1); electronics tester (1); lighted pliers (1); magnifier (2); pedometer (4); screwdriver (1); tire gauge (1)			
Miscellaneous	57	2.5	3.3
3-dimensional glasses (1); blanket (1); camera (1); coin storage machine (1); computer (1); computer mouse (1); cup (1); dog shock collar (1); doorbell (1); exercise device (1); fishing bobber (1); fitness tracker (2); flashing ball (1); guitar tuner (2); Halloween candy pail (1); headset (1); insulin pump (1); key finder (1); knitting or crochet needle (2); lighted ball (2); lighted balloon (2); lighted bucket (1); lighted candy (1); lighted cup (1); lighted notebook (1); microphone (2); mirror (2); musical magnet (1); night vision glasses (1); piggy bank (1); potty chair (1); potty timer (1); pumpkin light (1); rifle sight (2); safety flame (1); science kit (1); shirt press (1); snow globe (1); telemetry (1); timer (4); wireless keyboard (1)			
Music/media players	4	0.2	0.2
Ornament (including holiday decorations)	17	0.7	1.0
Pen	9	0.4	0.5
Phone, cell phone, or toy phone	10	0.4	0.6

(continued on next page)

Table 3
(continued)

Intended Use	Frequency	Percent	Valid Percent
Remote control (including garage door openers [4], TV, media, fan)	67	2.9	3.9
Scale	12	0.5	0.7
Thermometer	22	1.0	1.3
Watch	78	3.4	4.5
Unknown	574	24.8	
Total	2314	100.0	100.0

NEW BUTTON BATTERY DESIGN

Safer BB designs are being explored so they *do not cause injury* in the body. Quantum Tunneling Composite Coating (QTCC) has been reported as a potential solution. The QTCC is a pressure-sensitive coating. It has been shown in an in vivo model to render the BB nonconductive in the low-pressure gastrointestinal tract, but conductive in higher-pressure standard BB compartments.[31] BB design changes to render BBs safe within the body and their adoption by industry are critical to saving children from the associated morbidity and mortality.

Table 4
Intended use of ingested 20-mm lithium button batteries, July 2014 to June 2016: the top 3 product sources were remote controls, lights, and candles

Intended Use	Frequency	Percent	Valid Percent
Calculator	2	0.9	1.5
Candle (flameless, tea)	19	8.9	14.0
Car remote, key fob	6	2.8	4.4
Game/toy	18	8.4	13.2
Light	20	9.3	14.7
Book light (2); flashing ball light (1); flashlight (7); hat light (1); headlamp (1); keychain flashlight (1); night light (1)			
Miscellaneous	19	8.9	14.0
3-dimensional glasses (4); car alarm (1); Christmas ornament (2); cochlear implant (1); computer (1); dog shock collar (1); doorbell (1); fitness tracker (1); guitar tuner (2); key finder (1); lighted notebook (1); rifle sight (1); science kit (1); wireless keyboard (1)			
Remote control (including garage door openers, TV, media)	34	15.9	25.0
Scale	8	3.7	5.9
Thermometer	3	1.4	2.2
Watch	7	3.3	5.1
Unknown	78	36.4	
Total	214	100.0	100.0

Child with Non-Specific Symptoms
Fever, cough, sore throat, poor oral intake,
difficulty swallowing, wheezing
Unwitnessed, Unknown Coin or BB Ingestion

Rapid, Non-Invasive, Zero-Radiation
Coin-Battery Detector Screening
Primary Care Office
Emergency Department
Urgent Care

Expedite Diagnosis and BB Removal

Fig. 5. Clinical algorithm incorporating new screening coin-BB detector device.

NATIONAL RECOGNITION

The National BBTF was recognized with the 2017 AAP Advocacy Award for the efforts described in this article. In addition, related research from members of the national BBTF has been given the 2013 Chairman's Circle of Commendation Award (CPSC), 2016 Ellen Friedman Foreign Body Award (ABEA), 2017 Seymour Cohen Award (ABEA), and 2018 Broyles Maloney Award (ABEA).

SUMMARY

The severe risks of BBs to children have been well known for 4 decades. The National BBTF has put forth a multipronged approach in an effort to reduce the morbidity and mortality associated with BB ingestion in the United States. Given that BBs are ubiquitous in the household setting, it is critical that collaborative relationships are continued. The National BBTF is an open, public meeting platform that allows all key stakeholders to communicate. This ensures that consistent efforts are made in an effort to prevent ingestions and when they do occur, to expedite care, using the latest treatment protocols both before and after removal. Injury prevention efforts will continue until BBs are no longer a source of significant injury to children.

REFERENCES

1. History of battery invention and development. allaboutbatteries.com. 2011. Available at: http://www.allaboutbatteries.com/history-of-batteries.html. Accessed April 15, 2018.
2. Energizer. Battery history. Available at: http://www.energizer.com/about-batteries/battery-history. Accessed April 15, 2018.
3. Battery University. Types of battery cells. 2017. Available at: batteryuniversity.com/learn/article/types_of_battery_cells. Accessed April 15, 2018.

4. Battery Association of Japan. The history of the battery. 2016. Available at: http://www.baj.or.jp/e/knowledge/history02.html. Accessed April 15, 2018.

5. I.E. Commission. International Standard IEC 60086-2. 2001. Available at: http://www.iec.ch. Accessed April 20, 2018.

6. Völker J, Völker C, Schendzielorz P, et al. Pathophysiology of esophageal impairment due to button battery ingestion. Int J Pediatr Otorhinolaryngol 2017;100:77–85.

7. Samad L, Ali M, Ramzi H. Button battery ingestion: hazards of esophageal impaction. J Pediatr Surg 1999;34(10):1527–31.

8. Litovitz T, Whitaker N, Clark L, et al. Emerging battery-ingestion hazard: clinical implications. Pediatrics 2010;125(6):1168–77.

9. Litovitz T, Whitaker N, Clark L. Preventing battery ingestions: an analysis of 8648 cases. Pediatrics 2010;125(6):1178–83.

10. Galligan C, Morose G. An investigation of alternatives to miniature batteries containing mercury. Portland (ME): Maine Department of Environmental Protection (DEP); 2004. Available at: http://www.sustainableproduction.org/downloads/MaineDEPButtonBatteryReportFinal12-17-04.pdf. Accessed May 5, 2018.

11. United States Environmental Protection Agency. Mercury in batteries. Available at: https://www.epa.gov/mercury/mercury-batteries. Accessed May 5, 2018.

12. United States Environmental Protection Agency. Implementation of the Mercury-Containing and Rechargeable Battery Management Act. 1997. Available at: https://www.call2recycle.org/wp-content/uploads/ImplementationoftheMercury-ContainingandRechargeableBatteryManagementAct.pdf. Accessed May 5, 2018.

13. National Electrical Manufacturers Association (NEMA). Household Batteries and the Environment. 2002. Available at: https://www.nema.org/Policy/Environmental-Stewardship/Documents/NEMABatteryBrochure2.pdf. Accessed May 5, 2018.

14. Jatana KR, Rhoades K, Milkovich S, et al. Basic mechanism of button battery ingestion injuries and novel mitigation strategies after diagnosis and removal. Laryngoscope 2017;127(6):1276–82.

15. National Capital Poison Center. Button battery ingestion statistics. Available at: https://www.poison.org/battery/stats. Accessed May 5, 2018.

16. Jatana KR, Litovitz T, Reilly JS, et al. Pediatric button battery injuries: 2013 task force update. Int J Pediatr Otorhinolaryngol 2013;77(9):1392–9.

17. National Capital Poison Center. Fatal button battery ingestions. Available at: https://www.poison.org/battery/fatalcases. Accessed May 5, 2018.

18. Consumer Product Safety Commission. CPSC issues warning on button batteries. 1983. Available at: https://www.cpsc.gov/Newsroom/News-Releases/1983/CPSC-Issues-Warning-On-Button-Batteries/. Accessed May 5, 2018.

19. National Electrical Manufacturers Association (NEMA). Statement from the NEMA Dry Battery Section Regarding Ingestion of Button Cell Batteries. 2010. Available at: https://www.nema.org/Products/Pages/Dry-Battery.aspx. Accessed May 5, 2018.

20. Midgett J. U.S. Consumer product safety commission log of meeting. 2011. Available at: https://www.cpsc.gov/s3fs-public/pdfs/foia_buttonbatt03172011.pdf. Accessed May 5, 2018.

21. S. 1165 — 112th Congress: Button Cell Battery Safety Act of 2011. 112th Congress. 2011. Available at: https://www.govtrack.us/congress/bills/112/s1165. Accessed May 5, 2018.

22. Center for Disease Control and Prevention (CDC). Injuries from batteries among children aged <13 years—United States, 1995-2010. MMWR Morb Mortal

Wkly Rep 2012;61(34):661–6. Available at: http://www.cdc.gov/mmwr/preview/mmwrhtml/mm6134a1.htm#tab2. Accessed May 5, 2018.

23. Spinner J. Energizer charges into child-resistant packaging. Packaging Digest 2010. Available at: www.packagingdigest.com/packaging-design/energizer-charges-child-resistant-packaging. Accessed April 15, 2018.

24. Duracell Inc. Lithium Coin Battery Safety - Duracell. 2016. Available at: https://www.duracell-me.com/technology/lithium-coin-battery-safety/. Accessed May 5, 2018.

25. Energizer. Coin lithium battery safety. Available at: http://www.energizer.com/responsibility/coin-lithium-battery-safety/preventing-coin-lithium-battery-injury?page=register. Accessed May 5, 2018.

26. Anfang R, Jatana KR, Keith Rhoades MS, et al. pH-neutralizing esophageal irrigations as a novel mitigation strategy for button battery injury. Laryngoscope 2018. [Epub ahead of print].

27. Consumer Product Safety Commission. ASTM F 963-17 Requirements. Available at: https://www.cpsc.gov/Business–Manufacturing/Business-Education/Toy-Safety/ASTM-F-963-Chart. Accessed May 5, 2018.

28. Jatana KR. Oral presentation. Handheld metal detector: future technologies to detect esophageal button batteries and coins. Presented at the American Broncho-Esophagological Association Annual Meeting. San Diego (CA), April 26–28, 2017.

29. Russell RT, Griffin RL, Weinstein E, et al. Esophageal button battery ingestions: decreasing time to operative intervention by level I trauma activation. J Pediatr Surg 2014;49(9):1360–2.

30. Eliason MJ, Melzer JM, Winters JR, et al. Identifying predictive factors for long-term complications following button battery impactions: a case series and literature review. Int J Pediatr Otorhinolaryngol 2016;87:198–202.

31. Laulicht B, Traverso G, Deshpande V, et al. Simple battery armor to protect against gastrointestinal injury from accidental ingestion. Proc Natl Acad Sci U S A 2014;111(46):16490–5.

Preventing and Managing Operating Room Fires in Otolaryngology—Head and Neck Surgery

Soham Roy, MD[a],*, Lee P. Smith, MD[b]

KEYWORDS

- Airway fire • Endoscopic surgery • Head and neck surgery • Electrocautery
- Coblation • CO_2 laser • Fire safety

KEY POINTS

- Otolaryngologists are at highest risk of experiencing surgical fires and should be aware of the risks in every procedure.
- Fires occur when all 3 elements of the "fire triad" are in close proximity: flammable fuels, an ignition source, and an oxidizer.
- The 4 major procedures in otolaryngology with the highest risk of surgical fires are endoscopic airway surgery, oral cavity/oropharyngeal surgery, tracheostomy, and cutaneous surgery of the head and neck.
- Eliminating or decreasing one arm of the fire triad significantly reduces the risk of fire formation in the operating room.

For any fire to occur, 3 components must be present (the so-called "fire triad"): an ignition source, a fuel, and an oxidizing agent. Otolaryngology procedures pose the highest risks for surgical fire, due to the close proximity of these 3 components during surgery of the head and neck. Fires have been documented during tracheostomy, airway surgery, adenotonsillectomy, and skin surgery of the head, neck, and

Disclosure Statement: L.P. Smith is an Associate Professor of Otolaryngology at Hofstra North Shore LIJ School of Medicine and is Chief of the division of Pediatric Otolaryngology at Cohen Children's Medical Center and the North Shore Long Island Jewish Health System. S. Roy is Professor of Otolaryngology in the Department of Otorhinolaryngology—Head and Neck Surgery at the University of Texas Medical School at Houston, and Director of Pediatric Otolaryngology—Head and Neck Surgery for Memorial Hermann Hospital Systems.

[a] Department of Otorhinolaryngology, University of Texas at Houston McGovern Medical School, 6431 Fannin Street, MSB 5.036, Houston, TX 77401, USA; [b] Department of Otolaryngology, Hofstra Northwell School of Medicine, Cohen Children's Medical Center, Northwell Health System, 269-01 76th Avenue, Queens, NY 11040 USA
* Corresponding author.
E-mail address: SOHAM.ROY@UTH.TMC.EDU

face.[1-3] Surgical fire has also been reported outside of the head and neck region in association with cutaneous surgery, a risk that may be much more pronounced if supplemental oxygen remains free-flowing in an open system and/or if alcohol-based preparations solutions are used.

Although relatively rare in the setting of all surgeries,[4] surgical fires can occur with some regularity in the head and neck region. Surgical fire can have devastating consequences for patients and operating room (OR) personnel.[5,6] Surprisingly, surgical fire represents the second highest incidence of liability involving injuries during procedures with monitored anesthesia. It has been estimated that approximately 650 surgical fires are reported annually in the United States, and as many as 1000 such events may go unreported.[4] More recent data from ECRI estimates that of a total of 200 to 240 estimated surgical fires annually in the United States, 20 to 30 result in severe injuries, with 1 to 2 mortality events per year. Surgical fire represents a "never event" and otolaryngologists need to be vigilant to prevent this potentially devastating complication.

In 2008, the authors' group surveyed members of the American Academy of Otolaryngology—Head and Neck Surgery about their experience with surgical fires.[7] Of the respondents, 25% had witnessed a fire in the OR, for which the most common ignition sources were electrosurgical units and lasers. The frequency of fires was comparable in endoscopic airway surgery, oropharyngeal surgery, cutaneous surgery, and tracheostomy. Not surprisingly, the overwhelming majority of the events (80%) occurred in the presence of supplemental oxygen.

Growing awareness and concern about the potential for OR fire to occur prompted the American Society of Anesthesiologists to issue a practice advisory in 2008 regarding prevention and management of OR fires,[8] which was updated again in 2013 (**Fig. 1**).

HOW OPERATING ROOM FIRES OCCUR

To understand the mechanisms by which surgical fires occur, each element of the fire triad should be investigated along with its relationship to the others. In any OR, potential ignition sources include lasers, electrosurgical devices (traditionally electrocautery units), heated probes, drills and burrs, and fiberoptic light cables. Many devices and items typically found in an OR provide the fuel, which include endotracheal tubes, catheters, nasal cannulae, drapes, surgical sponges, dressings, ointments, alcohol-based skin preparation solutions, gowns and gloves, blankets, packaging materials, and even the patient's hair and gastrointestinal tract gases. The most common oxidizers in a surgical suite are oxygen and nitrous oxide. Nitrous oxide, when heated, releases potentially flammable oxygen. In addition, oxygen and nitrous oxide gases remain more dense than room air, allowing pools of oxygen to accumulate around the neck and under the shoulders during traditional head and neck procedures. During airway surgery, these gases can enable fuel to combust and burn more easily than in normal air.[9]

In the authors' initial series of studies, they tested OR drapes and towels to assess the risk of burn injury and fire formation with endoscopic light cables and the electrocautery unit ("Bovie"). In those studies, they found that although common drapes and towels did not ignite on fire, drapes melted easily in the presence of fiberoptic light cables and provided no significant protection against electrocautery burns.[6]

Eliminating any 1 of the 3 arms of the fire triad significantly decreases the likelihood of surgical fires. Multiple options have been investigated for eliminating an arm of the fire triad. The initial studies of oxygen requirements suggest that a fraction of inspired

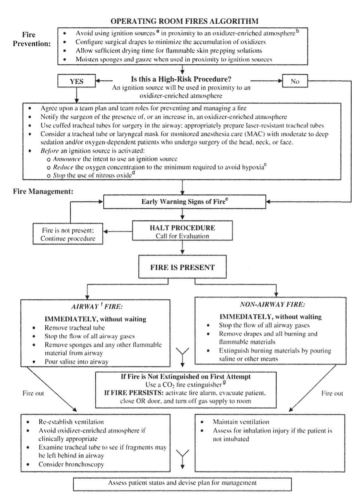

Fig. 1. Algorithm for management of surgical fires. [a] Ignition sources include but are not limited to electrosurgery or electrocautery units and lasers. [b] An oxidizer-enriched atmosphere occurs when there is any increase in oxygen concentration above room air level and/or the presence of any concentration of nitrous oxide. [c] After minimizing delivered oxygen, wait a period of time (eg, 1–3 min) before using an ignition source. For oxygen-dependent patients, reduce supplemental oxygen delivery to the minimum required to avoid hypoxia. Monitor oxygenation with pulse oximetry and, if feasible, inspired, exhaled, and/or delivered oxygen concentration. [d] After stopping the delivery of nitrous oxide, wait a period of time (eg, 1–3 min) before using an ignition source. [e] Unexpected flash, flame, smoke or heat, unusual sounds (eg, a "pop," snap, or "foomp") or odors, unexpected movement of drapes, discoloration of drapes or breathing circuit, unexpected patient movement or complaint. [f] In this algorithm, airway fire refers to a fire in the airway or breathing circuit. [g] A CO_2 fire extinguisher may be used on the patient if necessary. (*From* American Society of Anesthesiologists. Practice advisory for the prevention and management of operating room fires: an updated report by the American Society of Anesthesiologists Task Force on Operating Room Fires. Anesthesiology 2013;118(2):276; with permission.)

oxygen (Fio_2) of less than 50% may significantly reduce the risk of fire formation in open cavity surgery.[10] However, even at an Fio_2 of 50% oxygen, fire may still occur in closed-cavity situations such as endoscopic airway surgery.[11] The authors have also studied removing the source of ignition, because this may present the simplest option for reduction of OR fires. With this in mind, several experiments were conducted to assess the ignition risk inherent in 3 surgical modalities frequently used in ear, nose, and throat surgery procedures.

RISK FACTORS FOR IDENTIFIED HIGH-RISK PROCEDURES IN HEAD AND NECK SURGERY FOR SURGICAL FIRE
Oropharyngeal Surgery Including Adenotonsillectomy and Uvulopalatopharyngoplasty

A mechanical model of oropharyngeal surgery was created using a raw, degutted chicken. This cavity resembles the volume and size of a human oral cavity and oropharynx, and the organic tissue allows conduction of the electricity that powers electrocautery devices. A 6.0 endotracheal tube was inserted into the cranial end of the cavity and administered 100% oxygen at 10 L/min. The authors first activated an electrosurgical device ("Bovie"), and, subsequently, a bipolar radiofrequency ablation wand (Coblation) in the cavity. Each test was conducted for 4 minutes or until a positive result was obtained, and the trials were repeated to ensure accuracy. Ignition occurred, resulting in a sustained fire, after 25 to 80 seconds of use of the electrosurgical device. Neither ignition nor sustained fire occurred when the radiofrequency ablation (Coblation) wand was used. Pictures of these experiments may be seen in the work by Roy and Smith.[5] This experiment suggests that removing the ignition arm of the fire triad (electrosurgical unit) and replacing it with a nonigniting device significantly reduces or eliminates the risk of surgical fire in these types of procedures.

LASER AIRWAY SURGERY

Lasers used in laryngeal and airway surgery remain one of the highest risks for surgical fire in otolaryngology. In an excellent review of literature-reported cases by Day and colleagues, endoscopic airway surgery using laser surgery represented 25% of fires reported, second only to tracheostomy procedures, and lasers represented 17% of ignition sources in reported cases, second only to electrocautery units.[12] Others have studied airway fires resulting from CO_2 surgical lasers. In one case,[13] the CO_2 laser ignited a trans-tracheostomy tube during resection of a granuloma of the trachea. Another published report describes a fire involving an aluminum foil–wrapped endotracheal tube that was ignited by the CO_2 laser during laryngeal surgery.[14] It is imperative that otolaryngologists using lasers are very familiar with their properties and aware of the fire risk associated with their use. Lasers should be used with extreme caution in the presence of supplemental oxygen, even when using a "laser-safe" tube. Airway and oropharyngeal laser surgery should be performed either without an endotracheal tube or tracheotomy in place or with the laser-safe equivalent of those tubes.

Otolaryngologists must be aware that even so-called "laser–safe" tubes are still not completely safe. If the cuff on a laser-safe endotracheal tube is violated, the patient is at high risk for a surgical fire in the presence of supplemental oxygen.[15] Some otolaryngologists have advocated using wet pledgets superior to the cuff in order to minimize the risk of inadvertently violating the cuff with the laser. Data from the research team revealed that wet pledgets are not very effective at shielding the cuff of a laser-safe endotracheal tube.[11] Others have advocated double cuffed laser-safe endotracheal tubes where the superior cuff is filled with a liquid dye so that the surgical team is more likely to become aware if the superior cuff is inadvertently violated. With this system in place, the inferior cuff might stay intact preventing back leak of oxygen and minimizing the risk of fire. This seems like a more effective strategy then placing wet pledgets superior to the cuff of the endotracheal tube, although this risk reduction strategy has not been rigorously examined. The most commonly used laser-resistant endotracheal tube, the LaserShield II tube from Medtronic, is no longer available in the US marketplace.[12] There are currently 2 tubes available that claim a reduction in the risk profile for laser fires, including the Mallinckrodt Laser-Flex tube (a metal rein-forced, double cuffed tube) and the Rusch Lasertubus tube (a reinforced, single cuff tube). The otolaryngologist and OR team need to be keenly aware of the special risks associated with endoscopic laser surgery and the special steps that need to be taken to reduce that risk, including minimizing the Fio_2 during anesthesia delivery.

CUTANEOUS SURGERY OF THE HEAD AND NECK

Traditional transcutaneous surgery throughout the body should theoretically represent low risk of surgical fire, but transcutaneous surgery in the head and neck represents a much higher risk because of the close proximity of all 3 elements of the fire triad. Surgeons should be aware of the special risks associated with using alcohol-based prep-aration solutions for cutaneous surgery of the head and neck region. Although povidone iodine and many other iodine-based skin preparation solutions are not flam-mable, most commercial preparations involving chlorhexidine contain alcohol. Alcohol lowers the ignition threshold and supports combustion, easily igniting when touched with electrocautery to create fire. To minimize the risk of OR fire, surgeons should either avoid using alcohol-based preparation solutions when cutaneous surgery will be performed with an electrosurgical device or wait several minutes for the prepara-tion solution to completely dry before commencing surgery. Operating personnel are advised to consult the packaging on the individual preparation solutions to ensure that they are at least adhering to manufacturer recommended drying times. However, in one ex vivo model in the absence of oxygen, 10% of trials using alcohol-based prep-aration solutions resulted in a fire even when the manufacturer's recommended drying time of 3 minutes was followed; the risk may be even higher when the preparation so-lutions pool in low-lying areas. No fires were seen when nonalcohol-based preparation was used in the absence of oxygen.[16]

The risks may be even more pronounced when surgery is performed in the head and neck because of the close proximity of oxygen sources to the surgical field. The ge-ometry of the OR drapes and towels can affect the risk of fire because both oxygen and the vapors from flammable preparation solutions may collect in low-lying areas and underneath drape materials. Surgeons and Anesthesiologists should be aware of this concern and should arrange the drapes to allow for ventilation if possible. In addition, the use of a nasal cannula or face mask oxygen (open delivery system) allows free-flowing oxygen to serve as an oxidizer and when in close proximity to an ignition source (electrosurgical unit or laser) and flammable fuel substrate (alcohol-based preparation solution), serves to complete the fire triad.

As a result, current recommendations are that any surgery in the head and neck should be performed entirely without supplemental oxygen if the patient can maintain a safe oxygen saturation on room air. If supplemental oxygen of 30% or greater is required, it should only be delivered by a closed system (laryngeal mask airway or endotracheal tube), as stipulated by the ECRI institute and the Anesthesia Patient Safety Foundation in 2009. If oxygen is being delivered using an open gas delivery device (ie, face mask or nasal cannula), the oxygen should be discontinued several minutes before the use of a potential ignition source (ie, electrocautery).[17] In an elegant model of simulated facial surgery, a minimum distance of 5 cm was required during surgery with an electrosurgical device at 30 W and oxygen flowing at 2 L/min to prevent fire formation.[18] Indeed, in one closed claims analysis, surgical fires accounted for 17% of all claims associated with Monitored Anesthesia Care cases not involving a secured, closed airway.[19]

TRACHEOSTOMY

Fire during tracheostomy has been regularly reported and may occur under several different types of clinical circumstances, representing one of the most common causes of OR fires.[3,7,20,21] The most obvious scenario during tracheostomy involves an intubated patient receiving supplemental oxygen. Flash fire may occur if the electrosurgical device is used to incise the trachea or if it is used after the trachea has been incised, most commonly to cauterize any mucosal bleeding after opening a window in the trachea—a very hazardous occurrence, because the trachea at that point contains a column of oxygen and a flammable endotracheal tube in close proximity to the ignition source. Fire during tracheostomy may even occur if the tracheotomy is performed under local anesthesia with supplemental oxygen by an open oxygen delivery system (face mask or nasal cannula, as described earlier). The oxygen concentration can build up in the trachea while the patient is spontaneously ventilating, and there is a risk of flash fire if the electrosurgical device is used to open the trachea or at any point after the trachea is opened. The following steps are advocated to minimize the risk of OR fire during tracheostomy: (1) avoid the use of electrocautery to open the trachea, (2) perform tracheostomy using the lowest concentration of oxygen the patient will tolerate, and (3) avoid electrocautery after the trachea is incised if supplemental oxygen is (or has been) in use.

HOW TO PREVENT SURGICAL FIRES

The following are practical recommendations, based in part on the American Society of Anesthesiologists' practice advisory,[8] for the prevention of surgical fires:

- OR personnel should consider the risk of surgical fire before each surgical case. This may involve a "fire time out" or other standardized process; commonly used resources include the Christiana Fire Risk Assessment tool (**Table 1**). If a procedure is deemed "high risk" for surgical fire, the surgical team should formulate a plan outlining specific responsibilities for each team member to prevent a fire and for managing a fire that might occur.
- Because oxygen and nitrous oxide can contribute to combustion during surgical procedures, the anesthesiologist should collaborate with the otolaryngologist to minimize the proximity of oxidizers to sources of ignition (the authors' research suggests that a fraction of inspired oxygen [Fio_2] less than 50% may greatly reduce the risk of fire ignition in oral cavity surgery, but in the closed space of laryngotracheal surgery using lasers, even Fio_2 as low as 30% may result in fire[10]).
- With regard to cutaneous surgery of the neck and face planned under Monitored Anesthesia Care, when an ignition source is present, supplemental oxygen should only be administered in a closed system using either an endotracheal tube or a laryngeal mask airway.
- Because eliminating or minimizing any of the 3 arms of the fire triad may significantly reduce the risk of fire formation, the use of radiofrequency plasma

Table 1 Christiana fire risk assessment score		
Christiana Fire Risk Assessment Score	Yes?	No?
Surgical site above the xiphoid	1	0
Open oxygen sources (patient receiving supplemental oxygen)	1	0
Available ignition source (electrosurgical unit, laser, fiberoptic light cable)	1	0
Total score		

Score: 1, Low-risk procedure; 2, Low-risk procedure with potential to convert to high risk; 3, High-risk procedure.
Data from Medperts Medizinredaktion. Postoperative pulmonary complications. Medperts: Medical Experts Online. Available at: https://www.medperts.com/region/international/nephrology-blog?p_p_id=33&p_p_lifecycle=0&p_p_state=normal&p_p_mode=view&p_p_col_id=column-1&p_p_col_count=1&_33_struts_action=%2Fblogs%2Fview&_33_delta=20&_33_keywords=&_33_advancedSearch=false&_33_andOperator=true&p_r_p_564233524_resetCur=false&_33_cur=25.

ablation (coblation) in place of electrocautery or the CO_2 laser may significantly reduce the risk of OR fire. Both electrocautery and the CO_2 laser can cause ignition in the presence of an oxidizing agent and a source of fuel. The radiofrequency ablation device, however, does not seem to cause ignition even in proximity to 100% pure oxygen.

- Electrosurgical devices ("Bovie" or bipolar) should not be used to enter the trachea during tracheostomy (even if the procedure is performed under local anesthesia). Electrosurgical devices should also not be used once the trachea has been opened.
- Perhaps most notably, it has been the experience of both authors that almost every surgical fire resulting in litigation in the US stems from a lack of effective communication between members of the operative team. As they are frequently asked to review litigation cases around surgical fires, they have seen that almost every fire that is brought to litigation has one common theme: a failure of the surgeons OR staff and anesthesia teams to communicate in advance of the case to discuss the risk of fire. Commonly, surgical fires have occurred when the surgical and anesthesia teams have failed to ask about or identify the concentration of oxygen delivery before the deployment of an ignition source, resulting in a devastating fire.

The Joint Commission, a nonprofit group that accredits and certifies health care organizations in the United States, has also issued guidelines to help prevent surgical fires.[22] Specific recommendations include observing safety practices for the use of lasers, allowing patient preparation solution to completely dry before using equipment that can provide a spark, and minimizing oxygen concentration under surgical drapes. Iodine-based skin preparation solutions such as Betadine, contrary to popular wisdom, are not flammable. Chlorhexidine-based skin preparation solutions may contain alcohol, which significantly increases the risk of fire.

RESPONSE WHEN FIRE OCCURS

Every health care organization should implement procedures to ensure an appropriate response by all members of the surgical team when a fire does occur in the OR. The staff should act quickly and calmly to extinguish the fire and to protect the patient from injury. Three steps should be taken immediately and simultaneously: stop the procedure, remove the item that is on fire, and interrupt the flow of oxygen. If the surgery involves the airway or oropharynx, otolaryngologists should immediately remove the endotracheal tube and flood the throat with saline. These steps are critical for extinguishing the fire and minimizing patient harm. If the surgery involves the surgical drapes, all drape material should be immediately removed from the patient and away from the surgical field. Although it may seem that a small superficial fire has been stamped out, there may be a much larger fire under the surgical drapes. This algorithm is well delineated in the lower half of **Fig. 1**.

In order to increase awareness of the danger of surgical fires and to contribute to their prevention, any incidence of such fires should be reported to the Joint Commission, ECRI, the Food and Drug Administration, and state agencies.[10]

SUMMARY

Surgical fires represent a real risk and significant danger to patient safety. There are 3 essential elements required for fire formation, the "fire triad": an ignition source, a flammable fuel substrate, and an oxidizer. A systematic approach has been undertaken to study each of the arms of the so-called "fire triad" and determined that reduction of oxygen to less than 50% Fio_2 may significantly reduce the risk of fire. CO_2 lasers and electrosurgical devices such as the "Bovie" pose significant risk for fire formation, whereas radiofrequency ablation devices (Coblator) do not seem to carry the same risk. Careful attention to the inherent risks of fire in the OR and a team approach is critical in preventing serious harm from these potentially deadly incidents.

REFERENCES

1. Niskanen M, Purhonen S, Koljonen V, et al. Fatal inhalation injury caused by airway fire during tracheostomy. Acta Anaesthesiol Scand 2007;51(4):509–13.
2. Prasad R, Quezado Z, St Andre A, et al. Fires in the operating room and intensive care unit: awareness is the key to prevention. Anesth Analg 2006;102(1):172–4.
3. Varcoe RL, MacGowan KM, Cass AJ. Airway fire during tracheostomy. ANZ J Surg 2004;74(6):507–8.
4. Landro L. In just a flash, simple surgery can turn deadly. Wall Street Journal February 18, 2009. Life and Style, D1. Available at: https://www.wsj.com/articles/SB123491688329704423. Accessed September 12, 2018.
5. Roy S, Smith LP. Device-related risk of fire in oropharyngeal surgery: a mechanical model. Am J Otolaryngol 2010;31(5):356–9.
6. Smith LP, Roy S. Fire/burn risk with electrosurgical devices and endoscopy fiber optic cables. Am J Otolaryngol 2008;29(3):171–6.
7. Smith LP, Roy S. Operating room fires in otolaryngology: risk factors and prevention. Am J Otolaryngol 2011;32(2):109–14.
8. Practice advisory for the prevention and management of operating room fires. Anesthesiology 2008;108(5):786–801.
9. ECRI Institute. Electrosurgical airway fires still a hot topic. Health Devices 1996; 25(7):260–2.
10. Roy S, Smith LP. What does it take to start an oropharyngeal fire? Oxygen requirements to start fires in the operating room. Int J Pediatr Otorhinolaryngol 2011; 75(2):227–30.
11. Roy S, Smith LP. Surgical fires in laser laryngeal surgery: are we safe enough? Otolaryngol Head Neck Surg 2015;152(1):67–72.

12. Friedman AD, Gerber ME, Bhayani MK, et al. Ideal characteristics of a laser-protected endotracheal tube: ABEA and AHNS member survey and biomechanical testing. Ann Otol Rhinol Laryngol 2018;127(4):258–65.
13. Chou AK, Tan PH, Yang LC, et al. Carbon dioxide laser induced airway fire during larynx surgery: case report. Chang Gung Med J 2001;24(6):393–8.
14. Kuo C-H, Tan PH, Chen J-J, et al. Endotracheal tube fires during carbon dioxide laser surgery on the larynx – a case report. Acta Anaesthesiol Sin 2001;39:53–6.
15. Roy S, Smith LP. Prevention of airway fires: testing the safety of endotracheal tubes and surgical devices in a mechanical model. Am J Otolaryngol 2015; 36(1):63–6.
16. Jones EL, Overbey DM, Chapman BC, et al. Operating room fires and surgical skin preparation. J Am Coll Surg 2017;225(1):160–5.
17. Apfelbaum JL, Caplan RA, Barker SJ, et al. Practice advisory for the prevention and management of operating room fires: an updated report by the American Society of Anesthesiologists Task Force on Operating Room Fires. Anesthesiology 2013;118:271–90.
18. Reyes RJ, Smith AA, Mascaro JR, et al. Supplemental oxygen: ensuring its safe delivery during facial surgery. Plast Reconstr Surg 1995;95(5):924–8.
19. Bhananker SM, Posner KL, Cheney FW, et al. Injury and liability associated with monitored anesthesia care: a closed claims analysis. Anesthesiology 2006; 104(2):228–34.
20. Lin IH, Hwang CF, Kao YF, et al. Tracheostomal fire during an elective tracheostomy. Chang Gung Med J 2005;28(3):186–90.
21. Day AT, Rivera E, Farlow JL, et al. Surgical fires in otolaryngology: a systematic and narrative review. Otolaryngol Head Neck Surg 2018;158(4):598–616.
22. Preventing Surgical Fires. The Joint Commission. Sentinel Event Alert; Issue 29. 2003. Available at: http://www.jointcommission.org/SentinelEvents/SentinelEvent Alert/sea_29.html.

Reprocessing Standards for Medical Devices and Equipment in Otolaryngology
Safe Practices for Scopes, Speculums, and Single-Use Devices

C.W. David Chang, MD[a], Michael J. Brenner, MD[b],*,
Emily K. Shuman, MD[c], Mimi S. Kokoska, MD, MHCM, CPE[d]

KEYWORDS

- Sterilization • Disinfection • Patient safety • Reprocessing • Quality improvement
- Endoscope • Speculum • Medical devices

KEY POINTS

- Reprocessing standards for devices are primarily driven by assessed risk level to the patient: high-risk devices require sterilization, semicritical devices require high-level disinfection, and noncritical devices require intermediate to low-level disinfection.
- Flexible endoscopes used in otolaryngology are semicritical devices. Disinfection procedures depend on scope type and technique, with implications for adequacy, efficiency, and cost.
- Improperly disinfected or contaminated endoscopes can lead to disease transmission or even disease outbreaks. Individual packaging of speculums and related devices remains debated.
- Reprocessing of single-use devices is a highly regulated process requiring approval by the Food and Drug Administration.
- A nuanced understanding of disinfection/sterilization requirements and rationale ensure delivery of safe, ethical, and quality patient care.

Disclosure: The authors have nothing to disclose.
[a] Department of Otolaryngology–Head and Neck Surgery, University of Missouri School of Medicine, One Hospital Drive, MA 314, Columbia, MO 65212, USA; [b] Department of Otolaryngology–Head and Neck Surgery, University of Michigan School of Medicine, 1500 East Medical Center Drive SPC 5312, 1904 Taubman Center, Ann Arbor, MI 48109-5312, USA; [c] Division of Infectious Diseases, University of Michigan Medical School, F4007 University Hospital South, 1500 East Medical Center Drive, Ann Arbor, MI 48109, USA; [d] Strategic Partnerships and Innovation, Healthcare Quality and Affordability, Blue Shield of California, 50 Beale Street, San Francisco, CA 94105, USA
* Corresponding author.
E-mail address: mbren@med.umich.edu

INTRODUCTION

In the wake of high-profile incidents of patient harm from inadequate disinfection or contamination of medical instruments, reprocessing procedures have come under increasing public scrutiny, with a rapid increase in regulatory oversight. It has, therefore, never been more important for otolaryngologists to be knowledgeable and proactive regarding how medical devices and equipment are prepared for use in clinical practice. A variety of sterilization or disinfection methods are available, with the appropriate selection of procedure relating to type of device and its potential risk for infection to the patient. Adhering to approved and effective methods for reprocessing can ensure efficiency and mitigate liability risk associated with reprocessing. The delivery of safe, ethical, and high-quality patient care is predicated on a detailed understanding of medical device and equipment reprocessing procedures and their rationale.

GUIDANCE ON DISINFECTION AND STERILIZATION

Modern standards for disinfection and sterilization have largely evolved from the classification scheme introduced by Earle Spaulding in 1957.[1] Spaulding proposed the minimum levels of disinfection required of a device based on infection risk to the patient. Risk levels include critical (highest risk), semicritical (intermediate risk), and noncritical (lowest risk). Each risk level requires a different stringency of antimicrobial security—from simple disinfection to sterilization—that should be considered in when reprocessing such devices (**Table 1**).[2,3]

Critical devices, such as surgical instruments and implants, enter or encounter normally sterile regions of the body and are sterilized before use. The preferred sterilization processes include high-pressure steam for optimal inactivation of bacteria (including endospores), viruses, and fungi. For heat-sensitive devices, alternative methods include treatment with ethylene oxide gas and hydrogen peroxide-based gas methods. Liquid chemicals are a less attractive alternative, because chemically sterilized devices need to be rinsed and packaged in a manner not synchronous with actual sterilization, because the liquid sterilant must absent from packaging.

Semicritical devices contact mucous membranes or nonintact (broken) skin. Many rigid and flexible endoscopes used in outpatient otolaryngology clinics are semicritical items and thus candidates for high-level disinfection. Chemicals approved by the US Food and Drug Administration (FDA) for this purpose include glutaraldehyde, hydrogen peroxide, ortho-phthalaldehyde, peracetic acid with hydrogen peroxide, and chlorine (via electrochemical activation).[4] Rapid chemical reprocessing is practical for expensive, regularly used devices such as flexible endoscopes and inactivates most pathogenic microorganisms (viruses, bacteria, mycobacteria, and fungi); however, some bacterial spores may not be destroyed without longer exposure times.

Noncritical devices present the lowest risk to patients, because they only contact intact skin. Examples include blood pressure cuffs, patient seating and furniture, stethoscopes, and ear speculums. Intermediate-level disinfection is tuberculocidal, virucidal, fungicidal, and bactericidal but not sporicidal. Low-level disinfection is virucidal, fungicidal, and bactericidal, but neither tuberculocidal nor sporicidal. Intermediate-level disinfectants also provide efficacy against a broader group of viruses (enveloped and nonenveloped) and some mycobacteria. Examples include 70% isopropyl alcohol, iodophor and phenolic compounds, and quaternary ammonium compounds and are regulated by the Environmental Protection Agency.[5]

Table 1
Classification scheme for medical instruments

Spaulding Scheme	Otolaryngic Examples	Reprocessing Requirement	Bacteria			Fungi	Viruses	
			Sporicidal	Tuberculocidal	Bactericidal		Enveloped	Nonenveloped
Critical instruments Penetrate sterile tissue, enter the vasculature, or contact bone or blood	Surgical instruments, implants	Sterilization Steam Ethylene oxide gas Hydrogen peroxide gases	✓	✓	✓	✓	✓	✓
Semicritical instruments Contact mucous membranes or nonintact skin	Diagnostic flexible endoscopes, rigid scopes	High-level disinfection Glutaraldehyde Peracetic acid	Limited	✓	✓	✓	✓	✓
Noncritical instruments Do not directly contact the patient or only contact intact skin	Stethoscopes, patient furniture	Intermediate-level disinfection 70% isopropyl alcohol Iodophor and phenolic compounds Concentrated quaternary ammonium compounds		✓	✓	✓	✓	✓
	Floors	Low-level disinfection Diluted quaternary ammonium compounds			✓	✓	✓	

Data from Rutala WA, Weber DJ, HICPAC. Guideline for disinfection and sterilization in healthcare facilities, 2008. Atlanta (GA): Centers for Disease Control and Prevention; 2008. Available at: http://www.cdc.gov/hicpac/pdf/guidelines/ Disinfection_Nov_2008.pdf. Accessed May 19, 2018; and U.S. Department of Health and Human Services Food and Drug Administration Center for Devices and Radiological Health. Guidance for Manufacturers Seeking Marketing Clearance of Ear, Nose, and Throat Endoscope Sheaths Used as Protective Barriers: Guidance for Industry. 2000. Available at: https://www.fda.gov/RegulatoryInformation/Guidances/ ucm073746.htm. Accessed May 19, 2018.

OTOLARYNGIC ISSUES IN DISINFECTION AND STERILIZATION
Reprocessing of Flexible Nasopharyngoscopes

Most flexible nasopharyngoscopes are semicritical devices and should be cleaned thoroughly and at a minimum undergo high-level disinfection. Recommended reprocessing, detailed in **Box 1**, is a multistep sequence requiring attention to timely precleaning, leak testing, cleaning, disinfection/sterilization, rinsing, drying, and ventilated storage.[6,7]

Recent attention to sterilization procedures relates to infectious disease outbreaks traced to contaminated duodenoscopes, gastroscopes, cystoscopes, ureteroscopes, and bronchoscopes.[8] These scopes carry an increased risk if they encounter sterile cavities or have channels and ports that make cleaning and disinfection more challenging. In contrast, most scopes used in outpatient otolaryngology clinics have neither lumens nor contact with sterile areas. Nonetheless, some otolaryngology scopes used for sensory testing, laser treatments, and biopsy have lumens that may require more rigorous cleaning and disinfection processes. Channels should be flushed during the cleaning, disinfection, final rinse, and drying (with 70% alcohol and forced air) stages.

It is difficult to determine the risk of disease transmission from nonlumen nasopharygoscopes. Epidemiologic investigations are limited, because the detection of infection and linkage to the performance of an endoscopic examination is rare. No cases of human immunodeficiency virus, hepatitis B virus, or hepatitis C virus transmission associated with contaminated flexible nasopharyngoscopes have been reported in the literature. In a study where 1304 patients underwent flexible nasopharyngoscopy with improperly disinfected scopes, viral genetic testing was performed on 92% of these patients and no strong evidence of viral transmission was found.[9]

Endoscope reprocessing can be done by performing the steps manually or using automated systems. Manual approaches are susceptible to several pitfalls—human error, time pressure, disinfection liquid inconsistencies (inadequate monitoring of temperature, germicidal efficacy, and days of use), physical and chemical damage to scopes, and an inability to closely track. Automated systems cleanse, disinfect, and dry without human intervention, standardizing reprocessing and facilitating tracking. Damage to endoscopes is not entirely mitigated with automated reprocessors,

---

Box 1
Recommended reprocessing of flexible nasopharyngoscopes

1. Preclean the scope immediately after the procedure to remove bulk biocontaminants and prevent drying/hardening of debris.

2. Leak test the scope to confirm structural integrity.

3. Clean entire the scope with enzymatic detergent to remove debris and reduce microbial load.

4. Perform high-level disinfection or sterilization of the entire scope, including the handle.

5. Perform final rinse with sterile water or potable water.

6. Dry the scope fully.

7. Store by hanging scope vertically in a clean, dry, well-ventilated, dust-free area or cabinet.

Data from Muscarella LF. Prevention of disease transmission during flexible laryngoscopy. Am J Infect Control 2007;35(8):536–44; and Cavaliere M, Iemma M. Guidelines for reprocessing non-lumened heat-sensitive ear/nose/throat endoscopes. Laryngoscope 2012;122(8):1708–18.

because moving the process away from the clinic carries risks of damage induced by transportation and handling.[10] Additional disadvantages include the equipment and maintenance expenses, space required, cycling time, and volume limitations. Simpler systems automate only the disinfection step.

The use of sterile disposable sheaths has been described as an alternative to conventional flexible scope reprocessing. Sheaths cover the flexible tip and the portion of the scope that can contact a patient's mucous membranes, providing a contamination barrier between the scope and the patient. The FDA requires sheath manufacturers to instruct users to follow the cleaning procedure recommended by the endoscope manufacturer followed by intermediate-level disinfection such as wiping with a 70% isopropyl alcohol soaked gauze pad.[11] Studies have shown negative cultures on scope insertion tips after this procedure. Nonetheless, the use of sheaths would not prevent cross-contamination arising from a contaminated scope body or handle, from inappropriate technique in removal of the soiled sheath, or from soiling of a scope by a leaky sheath.[12] Because intermediate-level disinfection may be ineffective against endospore-forming bacteria such as *Clostridium difficile*, some investigators have advocated for high-level disinfection, even after sheath use.[4]

Storage and Packaging of Clinic Instruments

Traditionally, clinic instrumentation used in otolaryngology—nasal speculums, ear speculums, suctions, cerumen curettes, forceps—are stored comingled in an instrument cabinet. According to the Spaulding criteria, many of these instruments could be classified as noncritical, but some straddle the line between noncritical and semicritical. Short nasal speculums will only touch squamous lined vestibular skin at the nostril entrance; but, if inserted more deeply, speculums may touch intact mucosa, making the instruments' risk classification semicritical. Frazier suctions and forceps used during intranasal examinations routinely traverse mucosal borders and the devices are often used in nonintact mucosa as in nasal debridement procedures. Storage requirements for nonsterile but highly disinfected instruments may depend on the environment in which they are stored and accessed, because this influences the risk of cross-contamination.

A variety of potential sources of contamination are possible, although data on infection from office-based equipment are lacking. One possible source of contamination is medical staff, including the practitioner and support staff, when reaching into cart drawers with contaminated hands or gloves during a patient visit or between patients. Contamination may also arise from unattended patients rummaging through unsecured equipment cabinets. These concerns could be mitigated if instruments are stored away from patient access or contact. The Centers for Disease Control and Prevention guidance for packaging and storage of instruments is most explicit for instruments that must maintain sterility.[2] Approved packaging includes rigid containers, peel-open pouches, roll stock or reels, and sterilization wraps. Storage of semicritical instruments can be inferred from recommendations for endoscopes, which the Centers for Disease Control and Prevention simply states should be dried and stored in a manner that protects them from recontamination. Other recommendations suggest that the area should be dust free.

The Joint Commission has made a statement regarding storage of laryngoscope blades and handles used by the anesthesiologist during intubation, which may have bearing on otolaryngology practice.[13] The blades are treated as semicritical instruments requiring at least high-level disinfection. The manual goes further to state that the blades and handles should be wrapped individually and stored in a way that would prevent contamination. Examples include, but are not limited to, a peel packaging or containment within a closed plastic bag. Examples of noncompliant storage would include unwrapped blades in an anesthesia drawer, as well as unwrapped blades on top of or within a code cart.

Storage requirements for otolaryngology clinic instruments are evolving. Taking a cue from The Joint Commission requirements for laryngoscope blades and handles, some hospital organizations and accrediting inspectors now require individual packaging—including sterile peel packaging—of all instruments stored in instrument cabinets. Proponents suggest such practices decrease the risk for cross-contamination and allow for easy confirmation that instruments have been appropriately reprocessed and are ready for use. Detractors cite the lack of evidence demonstrating comingling and cross-contamination to be a clinically observed problem as well as the increased storage burden and inability to rapidly retrieve multiple variations of a desired instrument in an emergency. A recent study showed no greater culture growth from comingled instruments than peel-packed instruments at the end of a clinic day.[14] Again, it was noted that loss of efficiencies resulting from decreased storage room and increased difficulty in finding the correct instruments are also relevant considerations. This area awaits further investigation and data, but regulatory procedures suggest a growing trend toward increasingly stringent practices for individual packaging of office-based instruments in our specialty despite the lack of strong evidence to support this rigor. The American Academy of Otolaryngology-Head and Neck Surgery has had recent discussions with The Joint Commission to clarify this position. While still in evolution at the time of this manuscript's submission, The Joint Commission agreed that peel-packaging non-critical instruments is neither required nor expected. It was also agreed that such instruments may acceptably be stored co-mingled in clean cabinet drawers (personal communication). While we should pursue everything possible to secure the safety of our patients, it should be done to maximize societal good with responsible management of finite resources.

Reprocessing Single-Use Devices

Whereas most medical equipment was traditionally built for long-term use, the medical equipment industry and medical centers have come to embrace a wide range of disposable equipment. Disposable items do not need to be cleaned for reuse, reducing labor costs. Furthermore, high-profile reports of contaminated equipment and outbreaks of infection further fueled trends toward disposable equipment and supplies. Responding to market forces and incentives to minimize regulatory burden, manufacturers and health care centers have evolved toward a heavy reliance on SUDs.

Original equipment manufacturers (OEMs) decide whether to pursue single use or reusable classification for devices, but the standards are significantly more stringent for reusable medical devices. The OEM may label a device as single use when insufficient data has been found (or pursued) to ensure reusability. Because single-use devices (SUDs) do not need to meet these requirements, the cost of developing and producing SUDs is significantly lower than their reusable counterparts. Decreased production costs of SUDs and increased profitability of disposable devices thus create incentives toward single use labeling.

The proliferation of SUDs has tended to promote a throw-away culture in health care and an attendant increase in health care spending. Initially, the extra expense was passed on as a cost to third-party payers; however, this transfer of cost has become more difficult in recent years. As a result, the recurring cost of disposable equipment became a significant concern for medical entities. Faced with ever-tighter budgets, some hospitals had made their own foray into SUD reprocessing; this was relatively short lived, however, for a myriad of obvious reasons. The combination of liability concerns as well as the growing intricacy of reprocessing complex devices led to the development of companies specializing in reprocessing services. The use of SUDs not reprocessed in an FDA-approved manner violate sanctioned usage recommendations, which may violate public health laws and reimbursement allowances.

Regulation
The FDA is the primary arbiter of reprocessing standards. In response to growing concerns regarding the lack of SUD reprocessing oversight, in 2000 the FDA set forth policies and standards,[15] which were further fortified under the Medical Device User Fee and Modernization Act of 2002. SUD reprocessing companies are held to the same statutory and regulatory requirements of original equipment manufacturers. These requirements include device registration, quality reporting, and labeling. In addition to meeting all standards required of OEMs, reprocessors are required to submit a 510(k) marketing application, which provides data on the cleaning, sterilization, and performance of the reprocessed device. In addition, the device must retain reasonable quality to be substantially equivalent to the original after the maximum permitted number of reprocessing cycles.

The FDA categorizes medical devices according to a Code of Federal Regulations risk classification. It is this classification—which is distinct from the previously described Spaulding criteria—that dictates the specific requirements for reprocessing of a given device. Nasal cannulas, tongue depressors, and blood pressure cuffs are in the lowest risk category (class I). A variety of surgical devices used in otolaryngology are intermediate risk (class II). Examples include sinus microdebriders, harmonic scalpels, blades, bits, burs, syringes, masks, and some laser fibers. The highest risk devices (class III), such as coronary stents, heart valves, and implantable neuromuscular stimulators, are seldom reprocessed, although all are eligible for reprocessing. Although many class I and class II devices have received approval (**Box 2**), no class III devices have yet met the requirements for reprocessing.

Safety
The FDA stance is that reprocessed SUDs currently in use do not pose a safety threat. In the period spanning 2000 to 2006, there were 65 reports filed relating to reprocessed SUD, in comparison with 320,000 reports for devices overall. The adverse events involving reprocessed SUD were similar to those for new devices, but a comparative rate of device failure in reprocessed versus original products is unknown. The FDA concluded in 2006 that reprocessed SUDs were safe and effective options for clinical use.[16]

The scientific literature on the safety and efficacy of reprocessed SUDs is limited, with some studies suggesting decreased efficacy of devices or increased risk of contamination, whereas others show outcomes equivalent to new devices.[17–24] The variation within these reports may reflect variation in device complexity, design, and materials. Although some studies report on actual clinical experience, other literature involves experimental models. Given this paucity of data, clinicians who chose to use reprocessed devices in their practices should be conversant with FDA guidance on reprocessing and be mindful of the sterility and performance considerations of these devices.

Financial implications
The Centers for Medicare and Medicaid Services (CMS) and most commercial payers reimbursing for device costs do not distinguish between original SUDs and reprocessed SUDs. Because both are identified as single use, both are eligible for pass-

---

Box 2
Examples of commonly reprocessed single-use devices

Otolaryngology
   Coblators®
   Colorado microdissection needles™
   Adenoid blades
   Xomed shavers
   Harmonic focus®
   Ent shavers

General/gyn/urology
   Harmonic® scalpels
   Laparoscopic trocars and cannulas
   Scissor tips

Multi-department
   Pulse oximeter sensors
   Open/unused/expired items
   Somanetics®
   Neptune® manifolds

Orthopedic surgery
   Ablation wands
   Arthroscopic shavers and abraders
   Carpal tunnel release blades
   Athroscopic trocars and cannulas
   Drill bits and burs
   Anterior cruciate ligament blades
   Saw blades
   Rasps
   Tourniquets
   Reamers
   Scorpion needles
   ExpressSew™ needles
   Suture lassos, graspers, passers, and retrievers
   Countersinks

Ophthalmology
   Phaco tips

---

through payments, provided the reprocessing procedures conform to FDA standards.[25] CMS reimbursement generally provides payment for full procedures—not itemizing the individual devices—so there is the potential for significant cost savings. Similar considerations pertain to procedures in office setting or surgical centers, where the cost of devices is bundled into the facility expense component of relative value units for a procedure.

Reprocessed SUDs cost approximately one-half as much as original SUDs. Interestingly, the SUD reprocessing industry can put downward pressures on prices for original SUDs by creating competition in the health care marketplace. The Association of Medical Device Reprocessors reports cases in which OEMs have decreased their "rack rate" for new SUDs by up to 50% to compete for contracts.[26] As the business of reprocessing SUDs has grown, some OEMs have acquired the infrastructure to become reprocessors of their own products.[27]

Ethics

The subject of reprocessed SUDs has relevance to ethical principles of transparency, fairness, autonomy, and trust. 1 one perspective, the use of reprocessed SUDs is not off-label when issued by an FDA-approved third-party processor. The decision to use a reprocessed SUD with equivalent safety and performance profile to an original SUD might thereby be considered analogous to the decision to use any comparable instrument. Provided the FDA standard of "substantial equivalence" for reprocessed SUDs is consistently upheld, the decision to participate in a SUD reprocessing program is left to individual institutions. Informed consent does not typically involve conversations about the make or model of devices that a surgeon plans to use during a surgical procedure and it may suffice for surgeons to be knowledgeable and helpful in responding to patient queries on use of reprocessed SUDs.

One ethical consideration relates to potential asymmetric risk and benefit, wherein the patient primarily bears risk if a reprocessed SUD has impaired fidelity or residual contamination, whereas the medical facility enjoys the benefit of improved profit margin from cost saving on device and waste disposal. Respect for ethical principles is integral to the patient–physician covenant and delivery of high-quality care. The broad benefits of a greener health delivery system and reducing the overall costs of US health care can benefit patients, and revenue recovery from SUD reprocessing may allow hospitals to better fund quality and safety efforts or ensure adequate staffing. Nonetheless, these notions do not remove the need for transparency and careful reflection on this area. Any benefit to the environment or otherwise by adopting a "greener" approach is difficult to apportion to the patient, facility, or provider.

SUMMARY

Meticulous sterilization and disinfection procedures are necessary to ensure the safe and effective reprocessing of medical devices and equipment. Otolaryngologists should adhere to approved practices for endoscopes and other reusable devices. Practices continue to evolve regarding packaging and storage office based devices, with regulatory pressure increasingly driving individual packaging of nasal speculums and other contents of instrument cabinets without evidence to support these assertions. A rigorous, FDA-approved procedure also allows for responsible recycling of a variety of SUDs. Otolaryngologists' knowledge of best practice and transparency with patients regarding such practices ensure high-level care in the complexity of care we provide from various levels of devices. Future guidance should be refined to account for nuances in practice environment as well as the immune characteristics of the anatomic site where devices are being used.

REFERENCES

1. Spaulding EH. Chemical disinfection of material and surgical materials. In: Block SS, editor. Disinfection, sterilization and preservation. Philadelphia: Lea & Febiger; 1968. p. 617–41.

2. Rutala WA, Weber DJ, HICPAC. Guideline for disinfection and sterilization in healthcare facilities, 2008. Atlanta (GA): Centers for Disease Control and Prevention; 2008. Available at: http://www.cdc.gov/hicpac/pdf/guidelines/Disinfection_Nov_2008.pdf. Accessed May 19, 2018.

3. McDonnell G, Burke P. Disinfection: is it time to reconsider Spaulding? J Hosp Infect 2011;78(3):163–70.

4. US Department Of Health and Human Services Food and Drug Administration Center for Devices and Radiological Health. FDA-cleared sterilants and high level disinfectants with general claims for processing reusable medical and dental devices. 2015. Available at: http://www.fda.gov/MedicalDevices/DeviceRegula

tionandGuidance/ReprocessingofReusableMedicalDevices/ucm437347.htm. Accessed May 18, 2018.

5. US Environmental Protection Agency. Selected EPA-registered disinfectants. Available at: https://www.epa.gov/pesticide-registration/selected-epa-registered-disinfectants. Accessed May 18, 2018.

6. Muscarella LF. Prevention of disease transmission during flexible laryngoscopy. Am J Infect Control 2007;35(8):536–44.

7. Cavaliere M, Iemma M. Guidelines for reprocessing nonlumened heat-sensitive ear/nose/throat endoscopes. Laryngoscope 2012;122(8):1708–18.

8. Ofstead CL, Heymann OL, Quick MR, et al. Residual moisture and waterborne pathogens inside flexible endoscopes: evidence from a multisite study of endoscope drying effectiveness. Am J Infect Control 2018;46(6):689–96.

9. Holodniy M, Oda G, Schirmer PL, et al. Results from a large-scale epidemiologic look-back investigation of improperly reprocessed endoscopy equipment. Infect Control Hosp Epidemiol 2012;33(07):649–56.

10. Sowerby LJ, Rudmik L. The cost of being clean: a cost analysis of nasopharyngoscope reprocessing techniques. Laryngoscope 2018;128(1):64–71.

11. US Department of Health and Human Services Food and Drug Administration Center for Devices and Radiological Health. Guidance for manufacturers seeking marketing clearance of ear, nose, and throat endoscope sheaths used as protective barriers: guidance for industry. 2000. Available at: https://www.fda.gov/RegulatoryInformation/Guidances/ucm073746.htm. Accessed May 19, 2018.

12. Bhatt JM, Peterson EM, Verma SP. Microbiological sampling of the forgotten components of a flexible fiberoptic laryngoscope: what lessons can we learn? Otolaryngol Head Neck Surg 2014;150(2):235–6.

13. The Joint Commission. Laryngoscopes blades and handles - how to clean, disinfect and store these devices. Available at: https://www.jointcommission.org/standards_information/jcfaqdetails.aspx?StandardsFAQId=1201&StandardsFAQChapterId=6&ProgramId=0&ChapterId=0&IsFeatured=False&IsNew=False&Keyword=. Accessed May 19, 2018.

14. Yalamanchi P, Yu J, Chandler L, et al. High-level disinfection of otorhinolaryngology clinical instruments: an evaluation of the efficacy and cost-effectiveness of instrument storage. Otolaryngol Head Neck Surg 2018;158(1):163–6.

15. US Department Of Health and Human Services Food and Drug Administration Center for Devices and Radiological Health. Enforcement priorities for single-use devices reprocessed by third parties and hospitals. 2000. Available at: http://www.fda.gov/downloads/MedicalDevices/DeviceRegulationandGuidance/GuidanceDocuments/ucm107172.pdf. Accessed August 6, 2016.

16. US Department of Health and Human Services Food and Drug Administration Center for Devices and Radiological Health. Statement of Daniel Schultz, M.D., Director CDRH, Before the Committee on Government Reform - September 26, 2006. Available at: http://www.fda.gov/MedicalDevices/DeviceRegulationandGuidance/ReprocessingofSingle-UseDevices/ucm121067.htm. Accessed August 6, 2016.

17. Ledonio CG, Arendt EA, Adams JE, et al. Reprocessed arthroscopic shavers: evaluation of sharpness and function in a cadaver model. Orthopedics 2014; 37(1):e1–9.

18. Sabler IM, Lazarovitch T, Haifler M, et al. Sterility of reusable transrectal ultrasound transducer assemblies for prostate biopsy reprocessed according to Food and Drug Administration guidelines–bacteriologic outcomes in a clinical setup. Urology 2011;77(1):17–9.

19. Mues AC, Haramis G, Casazza C, et al. Prospective randomized single-blinded in vitro and ex vivo evaluation of new and reprocessed laparoscopic trocars. J Am Coll Surg 2010;211(6):738–43.
20. Lester BR, Miller K, Boers A, et al. Comparison of in vivo clinical performance and shaft temperature and in vitro tissue temperature and transection times between new and reprocessed harmonic scalpels. Surg Laparosc Endosc Percutan Tech 2010;20(5):e150–9.
21. Darvish K, Shafieian M, Rehman S. The effect of tip geometry on the mechanical performance of unused and reprocessed orthopaedic drill bits. Proc Inst Mech Eng H 2009;223(5):625–35.
22. King JS, Pink MM, Jobe CM. Assessment of reprocessed arthroscopic shaver blades. Arthroscopy 2006;22(10):1046–52.
23. Weld KJ, Dryer S, Hruby G, et al. Comparison of mechanical and in vivo performance of new and reprocessed harmonic scalpels. Urology 2006;67(5):898–903.
24. Roth K, Heeg P, Reichl R. Specific hygiene issues relating to reprocessing and reuse of single-use devices for laparoscopic surgery. Surg Endosc 2002;16(7): 1091–7.
25. Centers for Medicare & Medicaid Services (CMS). Pub 100-04 Medicare claims processing. 2015. Available at: https://www.cms.gov/Regulations-and-Guidance/Guidance/Transmittals/Downloads/R3425CP.pdf. Accessed August 6, 2016.
26. Association of Medical Device Reprocessors. The business case for reprocessing. Available at http://www.amdr.org/wp-content/uploads/2011/04/Business-Case-for-Reprocessing-for-web.pdf. Accessed August 6, 2016.
27. Stryker. Stryker announces definitive agreement to acquire Ascent Healthcare Solutions. 2009. Available at: http://www.stryker.com/en-us/corporate/PressNews/139133. Accessed August 6, 2016.

Publicly Available Databases in Otolaryngology Quality Improvement

Alexander L. Schneider, MD[a], Jennifer M. Lavin, MD, MS[a,b],*

KEYWORDS

• Quality improvement • Clinical registry • Administrative database • NSQIP • SEER

KEY POINTS

- Quality-improvement measures continue to take on rapidly increasing importance across all surgical specialties, including otolaryngology-head and neck surgery.
- Clinical registries are datasets that range in size from a few institutions to thousands of hospitals. They are populated by clinically trained health care professionals and data is collected with the goal of research and quality improvement.
- Administrative databases typically span thousands of hospitals and are populated by administratively trained billing professionals. They are maintained for billing and reimbursement purposes; however, their size and built-in infrastructure allow them to be used for quality improvement and research-related goals.

INTRODUCTION

The modern concept of quality in medicine was ushered in with the landmark Institute of Medicine's 1999 publication *To Err Is Human*,[1] in which it was described that at least 44,000 (and up to 98,000) yearly in-hospital deaths were attributable to preventable medical errors. Within the backdrop of the rapid expansion of focus on quality measures since the seminal publication mentioned earlier, the push for electronic health records (EHRs) began to take center stage. A 2005 article in *The Journal of the American Medical Association* (*JAMA*) "*Five Years After to Err is Human: What Have we Learned*?" prominently mentions EHR expansion as critical to advancing PSQI (Patient Safety and Quality Improvement).[2] A few years later, in 2009, it was clear

Disclosure Statement: The authors have no relevant disclosures.
[a] Department of Otolaryngology–Head and Neck Surgery, Northwestern University Feinberg School of Medicine, 676 North St. Clair, Suite 1325, Chicago, IL 60611, USA; [b] Division of Pediatric Otolaryngology–Head and Neck Surgery, Ann and Robert H. Lurie Children's Hospital of Chicago, 225 East Chicago Avenue, Box 25, Chicago, IL 60611, USA
* Corresponding author. Division of Pediatric Otolaryngology–Head and Neck Surgery, Ann and Robert H. Lurie Children's Hospital of Chicago, 225 East Chicago Avenue, Box 25, Chicago, IL 60611.
E-mail address: JLavin@luriechildrens.org

Otolaryngol Clin N Am 52 (2019) 185–194
https://doi.org/10.1016/j.otc.2018.08.004
0030-6665/19/© 2018 Elsevier Inc. All rights reserved.

that an essential component to improving on safety and quality was the provision and maintenance of standardized, publicly available, and, importantly, electronic sources of information spanning entire health systems.[3,4] Thus, the evolution of PSQI measures in health care has been wedded to advances in large, publicly available, electronic caches of data, or databases. The remainder of this article focuses on describing various publicly available databases used within otolaryngology head and neck surgery, dividing the databases into registries and administrative databases as can be seen in **Fig. 1**.

CLINICAL REGISTRIES: OVERVIEW

The American Academy of Otolaryngology Head and Neck Surgery defines a clinical data registry as "an organized system that collects uniform data (clinical and patient-reported) to evaluate specified outcomes for a population based on performance measures developed from Clinical Practice Guidelines."[5] Clinical registries typically contain data that have been collected and entered into the chart by clinically trained medical professionals who are familiar with the specific variables they enter into the data set. Registries are maintained for the purposes of research and PSQI. General advantages and disadvantages of clinical registries are outlined in **Table 1**.

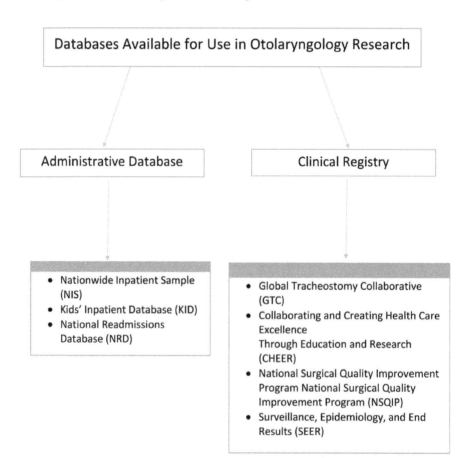

Fig. 1. Examples of clinical databases available to the otolaryngologist.

Table 1 Advantages and disadvantages of clinical registries	
Advantages	**Disadvantages**
• Created for the purposes of research/ improvement • Maintained by clinically trained professionals capable of accurately documenting pertinent patient-related information • Do not necessarily depend on *ICD-9* or CPT codes	• Costly to maintain from financial and time investment standpoints, as require their own separate infrastructure • Data collection slower than that of administrative databases • May be limited geographically, not able to extrapolate to the rest of the United States

Abbreviations: CPT, Current Procedural Terminology; ICD-9, International Classification of Diseases, Ninth Revision.

REGISTRIES: REG-ENT

One of the methods by which the Centers for Medicare and Medicaid Services (CMS) obtain quality-related data that drives reimbursements is from Qualified Clinical Data Registries that have been approved by the CMS. To that end, one of the more recent and well-publicized otolaryngologic clinical registries is Reg-ent, which was launched fully for the first time in September 2016.[6]

This registry is wholly electronically integrated for participating providers, remotely downloading information related to otolaryngology-specific quality measures in a manner that does not risk public health information.[5] The data collected in this registry were derived by the American Academy of Otolaryngology Head and Neck Surgery Foundation. The importance of actively defining what exactly otolaryngology-specific quality measures should entail has been highlighted elsewhere,[7] and this registry makes large strides toward that goal. The information in the registry can be used to compare individual performances with national benchmarks and could ultimately be used to drive research and clinical practice guidelines.

REGISTRIES: GLOBAL TRACHEOSTOMY COLLABORATIVE

Another clinical registry that is relevant to the practice of otolaryngology is the Global Tracheostomy Collaborative (GTC). The GTC, founded in 2014, is a multi-institutional and multidisciplinary organization dedicated to improving the care, safety, and quality of life of tracheostomy patients through standardization of care, education, and high-quality data collection.[8] It uses a prospectively maintained, validated electronic data capture system, REDcap,[9] to report data on tracheostomy patients, including demographics, comorbidities, surgical indication, death, accidental decannulation, tube obstruction, and bleeding.[10] A recent 4-institution study in the United Kingdom demonstrated improvements in tracheostomy-related care after enrolling into the GTC and reviewing the quality metrics it captures. Each participating site instituted measures aimed toward improving the quality of multidisciplinary tracheostomy-related care. Using the GTC database, there were significant decreases in hospital length of stay (LOS) and intensive care unit LOS as well as improvements in the time to initiation of oral intake.[11] In a single pediatric tertiary care center in the United States, participation in the GTC required minimal time expenditure and the record-keeping was accurate.[10]

REGISTRIES: NATIONAL SURGICAL QUALITY IMPROVEMENT PROGRAM

The National Surgical Quality Improvement Program (NSQIP) database was conceptualized in 1986, when the US Congress mandated that the Veterans Administration (VA) system report its risk-adjusted surgical outcomes compared with a national average. Shortly after its inception in 1991, there were sharp declines in postoperative morbidity and mortality in the VA system.[12] In 2002, the 3 private sector sites chosen to implement the NSQIP methodology published comparable 1 year results.[13] In 2004 the American College of Surgeons' NSQIP program was rolled out.[14]

NSQIP data are collected by intensively trained surgical clinical reviewers (SCRs), (typically registered nurses) who cull the information from the EHR and personally contact patients when necessary. Preoperative demographics, laboratory values, and comorbidities are collected, as are intraoperative data. Then, chosen 30-day postoperative morbidities and mortality are collected.[15] The SCRs use an 8-day cycle to select completed surgeries from their respective hospital's case logs: The first cycle begins on a given day, Wednesday, for example, and continues until the following Wednesday. The next cycle would begin Thursday and continue to the following Thursday. In this way, cases should have equal chances of being selected from each day of the week.[16] Each participating hospital assigns a surgeon champion to oversee implementation and quality initiatives. Hospitals are provided with biannual, blinded, risk-adjusted information to benchmark their complication rates and surgical outcomes.[17] In 2015, more than 600 hospitals participated in NSQIP; the inter-rater reliability for information abstraction from patient records was reported to be greater than 98%.[18] There is an NSQIP-Pediatric (NSQIP-P) that is predicated on very similar principles.[19]

The earliest publication in otolaryngology literature touching on the NSQIP database was in 2010.[20] Since that time, there has been drastic growth in related publications on a wide range of otolaryngologic topics: Of the 63 PubMed results when searching *NSQIP otolaryngology*, 47 were published from 2016 to the present. Interesting articles include comparisons in free tissue transfer outcomes between otolaryngologists and other specialties[21] and comparisons between thyroid surgery outcomes and trainee education between otolaryngology residents and other specialties.[22]

Limitations to the utilization of the NSQIP and the NSQIP-P for otolaryngologic research include the fact that it is a general surgery–oriented database: For the years 2009 to 2012, 1.2 million cases were captured, of which 2% were coded as otolaryngology primary.[23] Further, the particular postoperative events identified as complications by the NSQIP-P may not universally pertain to otolaryngologic surgeries, nor does the database allow one to evaluate outcomes specific to upper aerodigestive tract function. These concepts are well described in a recent publication using the NSQIP-P to evaluate pediatric airway reconstruction: Reoperation is a blanket variable within the database; therefore, planned bronchoscopy after airway reconstruction may be recognized as a complication by the NSQIP.[24] General cons include the fact that outcomes are recorded up to 30 days only and that only institutions that participate in the NSQIP are granted access to the data.

SURVEILLANCE, EPIDEMIOLOGY, AND END RESULTS DATABASE

The Surveillance, Epidemiology, and End Results (SEER) data set, managed by the National Cancer Institute, was created in 1973 and tracks data on patients with cancer from 18 geographic catchment areas around the United States, a population ultimately representative of close to 30% of the population.[25] Data points collected include demographics, tumor site, morphology, stage, and initial treatment. These data are abstracted from around the country from records originating from hospitals, pathologists, laboratories, health service units that provide treatment services (such as chemoradiation), and from those death certificates that list cancer as the cause of death.[26] In addition, each individual in the database can be linked to their Medicare claims.[27] The database is rigorously quality controlled, undergoing periodic case finding auditing by SEER auditors who verify that all SEER-eligible cases are included in the data set. Reabstraction is also performed, in which primary medical records are compared with registry records.[28,29] Since its inception in 1973 to the year 2015, the number of oncologic cases is greater than 10 million.[30]

In 2017, 40 years' worth of SEER data were used to explore the paradigm shift in head and neck cancer toward human papillomavirus–positive oropharyngeal squamous cell carcinoma (OPSCC). This study demonstrated that there has been an increase in the incidence of white men presenting with OPSCC and also showed that the rate of nodal-positive OPSCC increased as well.[31] Further, the database has been used to study patients with rare tumors, including head and neck rhabdomyosarcoma[32] and pediatric head and neck bone sarcoma.[33]

The SEER database is not without its limitations. Histologic information is entered into the database at the local level; there is no central review of histology.[28] Further, the nature of the geographic catchment areas make it such that urban areas and foreign-born persons are overrepresented.[34]

ADMINISTRATIVE DATABASES: OVERVIEW

Administrative databases contain large computerized data files that generally are compiled in billing for health care service, such as hospitalization.[35] There are many positive aspects to the utilization of administrative databases for research purposes. These aspects include, but are not limited to, the fact that the data are readily available in an accessible, electronic, and centrally stored format and oftentimes contain information related to comorbidities. They can provide detailed information regarding procedures, laboratory tests, and radiographic studies.

In many hospitals, the sequence of events by which information gleaned from the EHR is turned into part of the administrative databases is the following: Trained coders convert clinical information contained in the EHR, including the discharge summary, into numerical codes for diagnoses, procedures, and complications. This conversion is typically done using *Internal Classification of Disease* (*ICD*) codes. Subsequently, these codes are compiled into a discharge abstract, which is ultimately reported to state and federal databases that are in turn collated into large databases.

DRAWBACKS TO ADMINISTRATIVE DATABASES

Administrative databases come with their own drawbacks and challenges. The physical data itself are often stored in difficult-to-manage raw form.[36] In fact, *JAMA Surgery* has published a series of how-to articles regarding the best methods by which these large data sets should be utilized.[37] A 2017 *JAMA* publication further highlighted the difficulty in adhering to statistical soundness when using large data sets.[38] Secondly, as many administrative data sets are composed of records that were originally created for billing purposes, it has been proven some procedures are underreported (and, thus, inaccurately studied), as billing staff are financially disincentivized to record them.[39] With regard to the utilization of administratively recorded codes, the inaccuracy of *ICD* coding for particular patient characteristics, comorbidities, or complications has also been established in the literature.[40]

Herein the authors describe only a small sample of the administrative databases available to interested researchers, focusing primarily on the following data sets maintained under the auspices of the Healthcare Cost and Utilization Project (Kids' Inpatient Database [KID]) and the National Readmissions Database (NRD). General advantages and disadvantages of administrative databases are reviewed in **Table 2**.

KIDS' INPATIENT DATABASE

The KID is the only pediatric-only all-payer database sampling discharge data as described in the preceding paragraph in patients from birth to less than 21 years of age.[41] The KID data have been available every 3 years from 1997 to 2012, at which point 44 states were represented in the database.[42] The data elements contained in the KID include several variables specific to pediatric research: age in months for children 10 years of age and younger, designation of whether stay involved uncomplicated or complicated birth, and various hospital-level classification (pediatric, not a pediatric hospital, specialty pediatric hospital, or simply children's unit in a general hospital).[43]

Within pediatric otolaryngology and airway surgery in particular, the ability of the database to link charges to particular ICD codes has been used to study resource utilization and charges for rare entities such as laryngotracheal separations.[44] A 2016 publication used the hospital characteristics variable of the KID, showing that adenotonsillectomies performed in children's teaching hospitals were associated with higher costs and longer LOS but also that the patients in those hospitals tended to have more comorbidities.[45] Limitations of this data set include the fact that inpatient-only events are captured and repeat hospitalizations of the same patient will be captured as separate and unrelated hospitalization.

THE NATIONAL READMISSIONS DATABASE

Hospital readmissions have been estimated to account for as much as $17 billion in avoidable Medicare expenses.[46] Furthermore, in 2012 as part of the Affordable Care Act, the Readmissions Reduction Program was established. This program made it such that the CMS reduced payments to hospitals with excessive readmission.

The NRD is a database composed of data regarding all-payer inpatient hospital stays. When weighted appropriately, it contains information on approximately 36 million discharges from 27 geographically disparate states, accounting for 56.6% of all US hospitalizations.[47] Obtainable information includes standard demographics, *ICD*-based diagnoses and surgical interventions, payment source, and total charges.

Table 2 Advantages and disadvantages of administrative databases	
Advantages	**Disadvantages**
• Huge data sets provide ability to study rare pathology and can be weighted to represent the US population • Preexisting infrastructure that requires no maintenance on part of researcher • Built-in capability to study charges as were created for billings purposes	• Can be difficult to navigate • Coding by billers not uniform (financial disincentive to bill for certain procedures) • Billing staff not medically trained • Differences between what was coded and what clinically took place

Thus far, the handful of otolaryngologic publications using the NRD have dealt primarily with readmissions in head and neck surgery. Recently, head and neck cancer surgeries as a whole were analyzed using the NRD demonstrating a readmission rate of 7.7. It is expected that as familiarity with the NRD increases, the number of otolaryngologic publications related to this database will increase as well.

Limitations to this specific database include discrepancies between events that actually transpired in the postoperative period and the events captured in administrative databases. For head and neck surgery in particular, it is important to note that the NRD does not account for preoperative chemotherapy or radiation, factors that may lead to increased rate of readmission.

LINKING CLINICAL REGISTRY AND ADMINISTRATIVE DATABASE

As detailed in this article, neither a clinical registry nor an administrative database are perfect. A combination of the two may yield higher quality than one alone, as the scope and resource utilization information of an administrative database would be greatly enhanced with the clinical granularity a registry provides. This concept of integrating data sets has been successfully carried out on the institutional registry scale to evaluate postoperative readmissions, on the specialty-specific level to link administrative data with a thoracic surgery registry,[48] and on the national registry level whereby the NSQIP-P was integrated with an administrative database to explore health care utilization in the first year after surgery. The merging of clinical registry and administrative database remains untapped in the otolaryngologic literature and represents an exciting forefront in quality-improvement research.

SUMMARY

Quality-improvement research has fully taken center stage across the surgical spectrum, and otolaryngology head and neck surgery has been no exception. These efforts are inextricably linked with not only the betterment of patient care but also with appropriate reimbursement. Clinical registries that have been used within otolaryngology range from procedure-specific multi-institutional data sets (GTC) to those that span the entire country and hundreds of variables (NSQIP). Administrative data sets represent an exciting area into which otolaryngologists are rapidly expanding. A combination of the two should continue to be used in the years to come.

REFERENCES

1. Kohn LT, Corrigan JM, Donaldson MS, et al, editors. To err is human: building a safer health system. Washington, DC: National Academies Press (US); 2000. Copyright 2000 by the National Academy of Sciences. All rights reserved.
2. Leape LL, Berwick DM. Five years after to err is human: what have we learned? JAMA 2005;293(19):2384–90.
3. Clancy CM. Where we are a decade after to err is human. J Patient Saf 2009;5(4): 199–200.
4. Larkin H. 10 years, 5 voices, 1 challenge. To Err is Human jump-started a movement to improve patient safety. How far have we come? Where do we go from here? Hosp Health Netw 2009;83(10):24–8.
5. American Academy of Otolaryngology Head and Neck Surgery. Reg-ent ENT Clinical Data Registry FAQS. 2018. Available at: http://www.entnet.org/content/regent-ent-clinical-data-registry-faqs. Accessed May 15, 2018.

6. Sataloff RT. Regent: an invaluable new offering from the American Academy of Otolaryngology-Head and Neck Surgery. Ear Nose Throat J 2017;96(4–5):154.

7. Gourin CG, Couch ME. Defining quality in the era of health care reform. JAMA Otolaryngol Head Neck Surg 2014;140(11):997–8.

8. Global Tracheostomy Collaborative. Global trach about us. 2018. Available at: http://globaltrach.org/about. Accessed May 15, 2018.

9. Harris PA, Taylor R, Thielke R, et al. Research electronic data capture (REDCap)– a metadata-driven methodology and workflow process for providing translational research informatics support. J Biomed Inform 2009;42(2):377–81.

10. Lavin J, Shah R, Greenlick H, et al. The Global Tracheostomy Collaborative: one institution's experience with a new quality improvement initiative. Int J Pediatr Otorhinolaryngol 2016;80:106–8.

11. McGrath BA, Lynch J, Bonvento B, et al. Evaluating the quality improvement impact of the Global Tracheostomy Collaborative in four diverse NHS hospitals. BMJ Qual Improv Rep 2017;6(1) [pii:bmjqir.u220636.w7996].

12. Khuri SF, Daley J, Henderson W, et al. The Department of Veterans Affairs' NSQIP: the first national, validated, outcome-based, risk-adjusted, and peer-controlled program for the measurement and enhancement of the quality of surgical care. National VA Surgical Quality Improvement Program. Ann Surg 1998;228(4): 491–507.

13. Fink AS, Campbell DA Jr, Mentzer RM Jr, et al. The National Surgical Quality Improvement Program in non-veterans administration hospitals: initial demonstration of feasibility. Ann Surg 2002;236(3):344–53 [discussion: 353–4].

14. Velanovich V, Rubinfeld I, Patton JH Jr, et al. Implementation of the National Surgical Quality Improvement Program: critical steps to success for surgeons and hospitals. Am J Med Qual 2009;24(6):474–9.

15. Cohen ME, Ko CY, Bilimoria KY, et al. Optimizing ACS NSQIP modeling for evaluation of surgical quality and risk: patient risk adjustment, procedure mix adjustment, shrinkage adjustment, and surgical focus. J Am Coll Surg 2013;217(2): 336–46.e1.

16. American College of Surgeons National Surgical Quality Improvement Program. User Guide for the 2016 ACS NSQIP Participant Use Data File (PUF). 2017. Available at: https://www.facs.org/~/media/files/quality%20programs/nsqip/nsqip_puf_userguide_2016.ashx. Accessed May 30, 2018.

17. American College of Surgeons. About ACS NSQIP. 2018. Available at: https://www.facs.org/quality-programs/acs-nsqip/about. Accessed May 15, 2018.

18. Ottesen TD, Zogg CK, Haynes MS, et al. Dialysis patients undergoing total knee arthroplasty have significantly increased odds of perioperative adverse events independent of demographic and comorbidity factors. J Arthroplasty 2018;33(9): 2827–34.

19. Raval MV, Dillon PW, Bruny JL, et al. Pediatric American College of Surgeons National Surgical Quality Improvement Program: feasibility of a novel, prospective assessment of surgical outcomes. J Pediatr Surg 2011;46(1):115–21.

20. Stachler RJ, Yaremchuk K, Ritz J. Preliminary NSQIP results: a tool for quality improvement. JAMA Otolaryngol Head Neck Surg 2010;143(1):26–30, 30.e1-3.

21. Kordahi AM, Hoppe IC, Lee ES. A comparison of free tissue transfers to the head and neck performed by surgeons and otolaryngologists. J Craniofac Surg 2016; 27(1):e82–5.

22. Monteiro R, Mino JS, Siperstein AE. Trends and disparities in education between specialties in thyroid and parathyroid surgery: an analysis of 55,402 NSQIP patients. Surgery 2013;154(4):720–8 [discussion: 728–9].

23. Schneider AL, Deig CR, Prasad KG, et al. Ability of the national surgical quality improvement program risk calculator to predict complications following total laryngectomy. JAMA Otolaryngol Head Neck Surg 2016;142(10):972–9.

24. Roxbury CR, Jatana KR, Shah RK, et al. Safety and postoperative adverse events in pediatric airway reconstruction: analysis of ACS-NSQIP-P 30-day outcomes. Laryngoscope 2017;127(2):504–8.

25. Zhu VZ, Tuggle CT, Au AF. Promise and limitations of big data research in plastic surgery. Ann Plast Surg 2016;76(4):453–8.

26. Gloeckler Ries LA, Reichman ME, Lewis DR, et al. Cancer survival and incidence from the Surveillance, Epidemiology, and End Results (SEER) program. Oncologist 2003;8(6):541–52.

27. Lang K, Menzin J, Earle CC, et al. The economic cost of squamous cell cancer of the head and neck: findings from linked SEER-Medicare data. Arch Otolaryngol Head Neck Surg 2004;130(11):1269–75.

28. Scosyrev E, Messing J, Noyes K, et al. Surveillance Epidemiology and End Results (SEER) program and population-based research in urologic oncology: an overview. Urol Oncol 2012;30(2):126–32.

29. National Cancer Institute. National Cancer Institute SEER Training Modules. 2008. Available at: https://training.seer.cancer.gov/casefinding/quality/. Accessed May 16, 2018.

30. National Cancer Institute Surveillance Epidemiology and Results Program. SEER Incidence Data. 2017. Available at: https://seer.cancer.gov/data/. Accessed May 16, 2018.

31. Megwalu UC, Sirjani D, Devine EE. Oropharyngeal squamous cell carcinoma incidence and mortality trends in the United States, 1973-2013. Laryngoscope 2017; 128(7):1582–8.

32. Turner JH, Richmon JD. Head and neck rhabdomyosarcoma: a critical analysis of population-based incidence and survival data. Otolaryngol Head Neck Surg 2011;145(6):967–73.

33. Brady JS, Chung SY, Marchiano E, et al. Pediatric head and neck bone sarcomas: an analysis of 204 cases. Int J Pediatr Otorhinolaryngol 2017;100:71–6.

34. Foreword by Lazar J. Greenfield. In: Penson DF, Wei J, editors. Clinical research methods for surgeons. Totowa (NJ): Humana Press; 1987.

35. Iezzoni LI. Risk adjustment for measuring health care outcomes. 2nd edition. Chicago: Health Administration Press; 1997.

36. Johnson EK, Nelson CP. Values and pitfalls of the use of administrative databases for outcomes assessment. J Urol 2013;190(1):17–8.

37. Kaji AH, Rademaker AW, Hyslop T. Tips for analyzing large data sets from the JAMA surgery statistical editors. JAMA Surg 2018;153(6):508–9.

38. Khera R, Angraal S, Couch T, et al. Adherence to methodological standards in research using the national inpatient sample. JAMA 2017;318(20):2011–8.

39. Haut ER, Pronovost PJ, Schneider EB. Limitations of administrative databases. JAMA 2012;307(24):2589 [author reply: 2589–90].

40. Golinvaux NS, Bohl DD, Basques BA, et al. Limitations of administrative databases in spine research: a study in obesity. Spine J 2014;14(12):2923–8.

41. Lavin JM, Shah RK. Postoperative complications in obese children undergoing adenotonsillectomy. Int J Pediatr Otorhinolaryngol 2015;79(10):1732–5.

42. Tawfik KO, Sedaghat AR, Ishman SL. Trends in inpatient pediatric polysomnography for laryngomalacia and craniofacial anomalies. Ann Otol Rhinol Laryngol 2016;125(1):82–9.

43. Health Care Cost and Utilization Project. Introduction to the HCUP KIDS' Inpatient Database (KID), 2012. 2016. Available at: https://www.hcup-us.ahrq.gov/db/nation/kid/kid_2012_introduction.jsp. Accessed May 17, 2018.

44. McCormick ME, Fissenden TM, Chun RH, et al. Resource utilization and national demographics of laryngotracheal trauma in children. JAMA Otolaryngol Head Neck Surg 2014;140(9):829–32.

45. Raol N, Zogg CK, Boss EF, et al. Inpatient pediatric tonsillectomy: does hospital type affect cost and outcomes of care? Otolaryngol Head Neck Surg 2016; 154(3):486–93.

46. Jencks SF, Williams MV, Coleman EA. Rehospitalizations among patients in the Medicare fee-for-service program. N Engl J Med 2009;360(14):1418–28.

47. Health Care Cost and Utilization Project. Overview of the Nationwide Readmissions Database (NRD). 2017. Available at: https://www.hcup-us.ahrq.gov/nrdoverview.jsp. Accessed May 21, 2018.

48. Pasquali SK, Jacobs JP, Shook GJ, et al. Linking clinical registry data with administrative data using indirect identifiers: implementation and validation in the congenital heart surgery population. Am Heart J 2010;160(6):1099–104.

Moving?

Make sure your subscription moves with you!

To notify us of your new address, find your **Clinics Account Number** (located on your mailing label above your name), and contact customer service at:

Email: journalscustomerservice-usa@elsevier.com

800-654-2452 (subscribers in the U.S. & Canada)
314-447-8871 (subscribers outside of the U.S. & Canada)

Fax number: 314-447-8029

Elsevier Health Sciences Division
Subscription Customer Service
3251 Riverport Lane
Maryland Heights, MO 63043

*To ensure uninterrupted delivery of your subscription, please notify us at least 4 weeks in advance of move.

·

Printed and bound by CPI Group (UK) Ltd, Croydon, CR0 4YY

07/10/2024

01040505-0019